The Healing Power Of The Vagus Nerve

Guide to stimulation of the vagus nerve in the treatment of trauma with self-help exercises. Manage Anger, Depression, and Stress with Brain Therapy

Disclaimer

The information in this book is not intended as a substitute for the medical advice of physicians. The reader should regularly consult a physician in matters relating to his/her health and particularly concerning any symptoms that may require diagnosis or medical attention.

©Copyright 2019 D. Richard Scofield. All rights reserved.

This document is geared towards providing exact and reliable information with regards to the topic and issue covered. The publication is sold with the idea that the publisher is not required to render accounting, officially permitted, or otherwise, qualified services. If advice is necessary, legal or professional, a practiced individual in the profession should be ordered.

From a Declaration of Principles which was accepted and approved equally by a Committee of the American Bar Association and a Committee of Publishers and Associations. In no way is it legal to reproduce, duplicate, or transmit any part of this document in either electronic means or in printed format. Recording of this publication is strictly prohibited and any storage of this document is not allowed unless with written permission from the publisher.

All rights reserved. The information provided herein is stated to be truthful and consistent, in that any liability, in terms of inattention or otherwise, by any usage or abuse of any policies, processes, or directions contained within is the solitary and utter responsibility of the recipient reader.

Under no circumstances will any legal responsibility or blame be held against the publisher for any reparation, damages, or monetary loss due to the information herein, either directly or indirectly. Respective authors own all copyrights not held by the publisher.

The information herein is offered for informational purposes solely, and is universal as so. The presentation of the information is without contract or any type of guarantee assurance.

The trademarks that are used are without any consent, and the publication of the trademark is without permission or backing by the trademark owner. All trademarks and brands within this book are for clarifying purposes only and are the owned by the owners themselves, not affiliated with this document.

Table of Contents

Introduction 9

What Is The Vagus Nerve? 13

Vagus Nerve Stimulation 24

Psychophysiology 35

Understanding The Psycho-Emotional Roots Of Disease 46

How To Strengthen Your Vagus Nerve To Upgrade Your Whole Body 57

The Polivagal Theory 74

Why Vagal Tone Matters 92

An Introduction To The Nervous System 104

Vagus Nerve Dysfunctions And Associated Diseases 140

Vagus Nerve And Anxiety 155

Depression (Major Depressive Disorder) 164

Vagus Nerve In Meditation 174

Physiological Benefits Of Meditation 182

Vagus Nerve Exercises 191

Method To Activate Vagus Nerve 198

Sound Therapy As Medicine To Stimulate The Vagus Nerve 210

Importance Of The Vagus Nerve For Health And Weight Loss 216

Conclusions 224

References 227

INTRODUCTION

The vagus nerve of the central nerve center is the commander-in-chief and manages all the major organs. This is the longest cranial ever to begin right behind the brain's eyes and interact with all of the body's major organs. This sends fibers from your nervous system to all your visceral organs and is the supervisor of your inner nerve center, delivering nerve impulses to each organ in your body. The term vagus means "wanderer" as it wanders throughout the body from the brain to the reproductive organs, touching all in between. When it comes to mind-body communication, the vagus nerve is important because it enters all the main organs except the adrenal and thyroid glands.

Anxiety and depression can be suppressed by the mind. The reason they communicate with each other is closely connected to the vagus nerve as it is connected to the nerves that guide our ears for speech, keeping eye contact, and those that control emotions. This nerve can also affect the proper release of hormones in the body to maintain healthy mental and physical systems.

It is the nerve that is responsible for increasing stomach acidity and digestive juice secretion for ease of digestion. When stimulated, it can also help to absorb vitamin B12. If it does not work properly, you may suspect, to name a few, severe intestinal problems such as colitis, IBS, and Reflux. Problems with reflux are triggered by a vagus nerve disorder as it also affects the esophagus. It is the inappropriate reflex of the esophagus that triggers disorders like Gerd and Reflux.

Also, the vagus nerve helps control blood pressure and heart rate, stopping heart disease. While this nerve regulates the balance of blood glucose in the liver and pancreas to avoid diabetes, the vagus nerve helps release bile through the gallbladder, which lets the body remove contaminants and break down fat. This nerve stimulates general kidney function while in the bladder, increasing blood flow, maximizing the bodies' filtration.

Activation in all target organs can reduce inflammation when the vagus nerve reaches the spleen. Even this nerve can control the fertility and orgasms of women. A damaged or blocked vagus nerve may cause havoc in the mind and body as a whole.

Now that we realize that the vagus nerve is connected to all the major organs and their proper functioning, we can easily conclude that any disease, infection, or brain, heart, and spirit can be reversed or even healed by triggering and relaxing the vagus nerve. So you're also going to have positive effects on issues like anxiety disorders, heart disease, headaches and migraines, fibromyalgia, alcohol addiction, breathing, gut problems, memory problems, mood disorders, and cancer.

There are many recorded ways to activate the vagus ' nerve, such as singing and humming, laughing, yoga, awareness, breathing exercises, physical activity, and vibration, to name just a few.

Singing and laughing stimulate the muscles on the back of your throat that stimulate the nerve. Also, mild exercise or rehabilitation raises the stomach fluid, which means activating the vagus nerve. A regimented yoga practice can also improve the activation of this nerve because of the motions, but relaxation help stimulate the nerve of the vagus.

WHAT IS THE VAGUS NERVE?

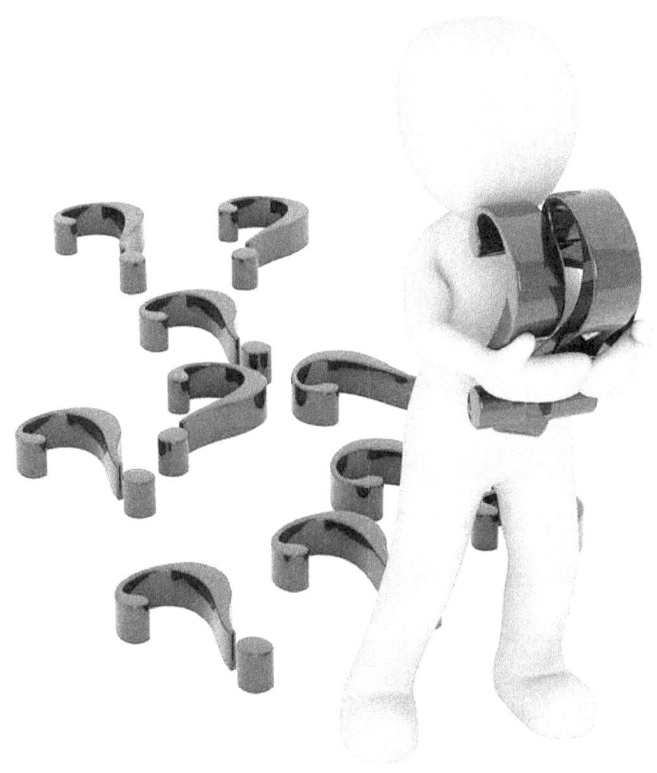

The vagus nerve, historically referred to as the Pneumogastric nerve, is the tenth cranial nerve and interfaces with the heart, lungs, and digestive tract part sympathy control. The vagus nerves are paired, but in the singular, they are usually referred to. It is the longest nerve of the human body's autonomous nervous system. The end of the vagus nerve is known as the nucleus of the spinal accessory.

Bidirectional communication between the brain and the gastrointestinal tract, the so-called "heart-good axis," is based on a complex system, including the vagus nerve, but also sympathetic (e.g. through the prevertebral ganglia), endocrine, digestive, and humoral relations, as well as the role of gut microbiota to control gastrointestinal homeostasis and link emotional and cognitive homeostasis. Over 30 neurotransmitters are produced by the ENS and have more neurons than the spine. Hormones and peptides released by the ENS into the bloodstream cross the blood-brain barrier (e.g., gherkin) and can act synergistically with the vagus nerve to regulate food intake and appetite, for example. As a treatment target of gastrointestinal and psychiatric disorders such as inflammatory bowel disease (IBD), anxiety, and post-traumatic stress disorder (PTSD), the brain-good axis is becoming increasingly important. The gut is an essential immune system control center and the immune modulator property of the vagus nerve.

As a consequence, this nerve plays significant roles in the gut, heart, and inflammatory relationship. For starters, vagus nerve stimulation (VNS), or meditation techniques, there are new treatment approaches to modulate the brain–good axis. For mood and anxiety problems, but also in other conditions associated with increased inflammation, these therapies are effective. Especially in both irritable bowel syndrome and IBD, gut-directed hypnotherapy is effective. Finally, the vagus nerve is also an important connection between nutrition and psychiatric, neurological and inflammatory diseases.

Introduction

Vagus nerve stimulation (VNS) is a neurostimulation procedure in which the vagus nerve is activated in the neck area through a helical electrode wounded around the cervical vagus fibers and attached to a lead to a sub-clavicular inserted pulse generator. It has become a valuable option for patients with refractory epilepsy in the therapeutic armamentarium over the past two decades and is currently routinely available in epilepsy centers around the world. Extensive evidence is also available in treatment-resistant depression for the application of invasive VNS therapy. Small studies and case study series have shown the efficacy of intrusive VNS in treating refractory migraine and cluster headache, Alzheimer's disease, anxiety disorders resistant to medication, bipolar disorder, and obesity. To improve efficacy and safety, numerous VNS instruments have been developed over the years. They will discuss the latest advances in invasive VNS technology for the treatment of epilepsy, more recently developed invasive VNS devices for other uses than systems for epilepsy and anxiety, and non-invasive vagus nerve stimulation.

The vagus nerve is the main component of the parasympathetic nervous system, which controls a wide range of vital body functions, including attitude regulation, immune response, metabolism, and heart rate. This creates one of the connections between the brain and the gastrointestinal tract and sends information to the brain through afferent fibers about the state of the internal organs. In this review article, we discuss various vagus nerve roles that make it an attractive target for the treatment of psychological and gastrointestinal disorders. There is preliminary evidence that activation of the vagus nerve is a promising potential therapy for medication-refractory anxiety, posttraumatic stress disorder and inflammatory disease of the intestine.

Treatments targeting the vagus nerve increase the vagal tone and inhibit the production of cytokine. Both are important resistance mechanisms. Stimulating vagal afferent fibers in the intestine affects monoaminergic brain networks in the brain stem that play critical roles in various psychiatric conditions, such as mood and anxiety. In row, there is preliminary evidence that intestinal bacteria have beneficial effects on mood and anxiety, in part by influencing the vagus nerve activity. Since the vagal tone is correlated with the ability to regulate stress responses and can be influenced by breathing, its growth through meditation and yoga is likely to contribute to resilience and mitigation of symptoms of mood and anxiety.

Basic Anatomy of Vagus Nerve

The vagus nerve carries the brain and vice versa with a wide range of signals from the digestive system and organs. It is the tenth cranial nerve that passes through the neck and thorax to the abdomen from its source in the brainstem. It was also described as the "wanderer nerve" because of its long path through the human body.

The vagus nerve exits in the groove between the olive and the inferior peduncle of the cerebella from the medulla oblongata, leaving the skull through the jugular foramen's middle compartment. The vagus nerve in the neck gives essential innervations to most pharynx and larynx muscles that are responsible for swallowing and vocalization. It provides the heart with the main parasympathetic supply in the thorax and stimulates a heart rate reduction. The vagus nerve regulates smooth muscle movement and glandular secretion in the intestines. Preganglionic neurons of vagal efferent fibers emerge from the vagus nerve's dorsal motor nucleus in the medulla and are external to the muscle and mucosal layers of the gut in both the lamina propria and the muscle.

The celiac branch supplies the intestine to the distal part of the descending colon from the proximal duodenum. The gastrointestinal vagal afferents include in the esophagus, stomach, and proximal small intestine mucosal mechanoreceptors, chemoreceptors, and stress receptors, and sensory endings in the liver and pancreas.

Vagus nerve dysfunction can lead to a whole range of problems, including obesity, bradycardia (abnormally slow heartbeat), swallowing difficulties, gastrointestinal diseases, fainting, mood disorders, B12 deficiency, chronic inflammation, impaired cough, and seizures. In the meantime, vagus nerve stimulation has been shown to improve conditions like:

- Anxiety disorder
- Cardiovascular disease
- Tinnitus
- Diabetes
- Alcohol addiction
- Alzheimer's disease
- Leaky gut
- Poor breathing
- Stress disorder
- Cancer

Structure

After leaving the medulla oblongata between the pyramid and the lower peduncle of the cerebellum, the vagus nerve extends through the jugular foramen, and then passes through the carotid sheath between the inner carotid artery and the inner jugular vein to the neck, chest and abdomen, where it contributes to the viscera's innervations and reaches the colon. In addition to giving some output to different organs, the vagus nerve comprises between 80% and 90% of afferent nerves, mostly transmitting sensory information about the state of the organs of the body to the central nervous system. The nerves of the right and left vagus descend through the jugular foramina from the cranial vault, entering the carotid sheath between the inner and outer carotid arteries, and proceeding laterally to the main carotid artery. The cell bodies of the vagus nerve's visceral afferent fibers are bilaterally situated in the vagus nerve's lower ganglion (no dosage ganglia).

The right vagus nerve produces the right recurrent laryngeal nerve, which loops around the right subclavian artery and ascends between the trachea and the esophagus into the chest. Then the right vagus crosses anterior to the right subclavian artery, runs back to the upper vena cava, descends back to the right main bronchus, and contributes to cardiac, pulmonary, and esophageal plexus. In the lower part of the esophagus it forms the posterior vagal trunk and enters the diaphragm through the hiatus of the esophagus.

The left vagus nerve crosses and descends on the aortic arch into the thorax between the left popular carotid artery and the left subclavian artery. It creates the left recurrent laryngeal nerve that hooks to the left of the ligamentum arteriosum around the aortic arch and ascends between the trachea and the esophagus. Therefore, the left vagus gives off thoracic cardiac branches, splits into the pulmonary plexus, proceeds into the esophageal plexus, and enters the abdomen as the posterior vagal trunk in the diaphragm's esophageal pause.

- the pharyngeal nerve
- the superior laryngeal nerve
- the superior cervical cardiac branches of the vagus nerve
- the lower cervical cardiac branch
- the recurrent laryngeal nerve

- the thoracic cardiac branches
- the pulmonary plexus branches
- the esophageal plexus branches
- the anterior vagal trunk
- the posterior vagal trunk

The vagus passes in the carotid sheath perpendicular to the common carotid artery and the internal jugular vein.

VAGUS NERVE STIMULATION

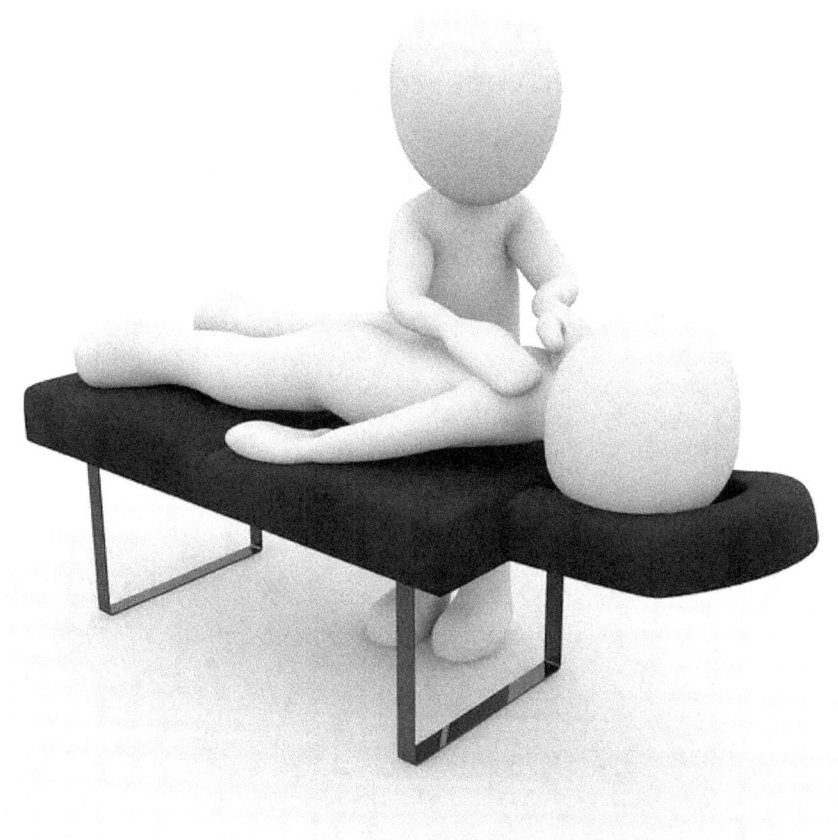

Stimulation of the vagus nerve requires the use of a system of electrical impulses to activate the vagus nerve. For the treatment of epilepsy and anxiety, an implantable vagus nerve stimulator is currently approved by the FDA.

On each side of your body, there is one vagus nerve flowing from your brainstem to your chest and abdomen through your head.

A machine is surgically implanted in your chest under the skin for traditional vagus nerve stimulation, and a tube is threaded under your skin linking the device to the left vagus nerve. The system delivers electrical signals to your brainstem if triggered along the left vagus nerve, which then sends signals to certain parts of your brain. The right vagus nerve is not used because fibers that supply nerves to the heart are more likely to be carried.

Advanced, non-invasive products for vagus nerve stimulation that do not require surgical implantation have been approved for the treatment of anxiety, insomnia and pain in Europe. The Food and Drug Administration recently approved a non-invasive device that activates the vagus nerve to treat cluster headaches in the United States.

Why it's achieved

About one-third of people with epilepsy are not responding entirely to anti-seizure medications. Stimulation of the vagus nerve may be an alternative to reduce the occurrence of seizures in patients who have not gained drug regulation.

Vagus nerve stimulation may also be helpful for people who have not progressed to intense treatments for depression, such as antidepressant drugs, psychological counselling (psychotherapy) or electroconvulsive therapy (ECT).

Vagus nerve stimulation has been approved by the Food and Drug Administration (FDA) for patients who:

- Are four years of age or older
- Have focal (partial) epilepsy
- Have hallucinations with drugs that are not well controlled.

The FDA has licensed vagus nerve stimulation for the treatment of depression for adolescents who:

- Experience chronic, hard-to-treat depression (treatment-resistant depression)
- Have not progressed after four or more medications and electroconvulsive therapy (ECT) have been tried, or both
- Practice traditional depression therapies along with vagus nerve stimulation.

Risks

Stimulation of the vagus nerve is healthy for most individuals. But it does have many complications, from both the device's surgery to insert and the activation of the brain.

Surgery risks

Surgical complications of activation of the inserted vagus nerve are uncommon and comparable to those of other forms of surgery. These include:

- Cutting pressure (incision) to insert the tool

- Infection
- Swallowing trouble
- Paralysis of the vocal cord, which is usually temporary but may be permanent

Side effects after surgery

Some of the side effects and health problems associated with implanted nerve stimulation may include:

Voice changes

- Hoarseness
- Throat pressure
- Cough
- Headaches
- Shortness of breath
- Difficulty swallowing
- Skin tingling and prickling
- Insomnia
- Sleep apnea worsening

Side effects are tolerable for most individuals. These can decrease over time, but for as long as you use embedded vagus nerve stimulation, certain side effects can stay irritating.

Such effects can be reduced by changing the electrical impulses. The system can be turned down temporarily or permanently when side effects are unacceptable.

How to prepare

Before you agree to have the treatment, it is important to consider carefully the pros and cons of implanted vagus nerve stimulation. Make sure you know what all your other treatment options are, and both of you and your doctor agree that the best option for you is artificial vagus nerve stimulation. Ask your doctor exactly what to expect during surgery and after the pulse generator has been installed.

Food and medications

You may need to stop taking some drugs in advance and may ask your doctor not to eat the night before the operation.

Before the procedure, your doctor will perform a physical examination. You may need blood tests or other tests to make sure you have no health concerns that could be an issue. Until surgery, the doctor may have you begin to take antibiotics to prevent infection.

During the procedure

Surgery can be conducted on an outpatient basis to implant the vagus nerve stimulation device, although some doctors prefer that you stay overnight.

Generally, the procedure takes an hour to an hour and a half. You may stay awake, but have medicine to relax the surgical region (local anesthesia), or you may be asleep during the procedure (general anesthesia).

The brain is not involved in the surgery itself. There are two incisions, one on the chest or in the axillary area, and the other on the left side of the neck.

The pulse generator is located on your chest's upper left side. The system was supposed to be a permanent implant, but if necessary, it can be removed.

The pulse generator runs on battery power and is about the size of a stopwatch. The pulse generator is attached to a lead cable. The lead wire is directed from your abdomen to your neck under your hair, where it is threaded through the second incision to the left vagus nerve.

After the procedure

During a visit to your doctor's office a few weeks after surgery, the pulse generator is turned on. Then it can be programmed at different durations, frequencies and currents to transmit electrical impulses to the vagus nerve. Based on your signs and side effects, vagus nerve stimulation usually begins at a low level and is gradually increased.

During different intervals, activation is designed to turn on and off— like 30 seconds on, five minutes off. When the nerve stimulation is on, you may have some tingling feelings and mild pain in your neck or occasional heaviness.

The stimulator does not trigger signs of epilepsy or anxiety. Once powered on, the simulator will turn on and off at the doctor's specified times. For example, when you sense an approaching seizure, you can use a hand-held magnet to induce relaxation at a different time.

The magnet can also be used to briefly shut off the activation of the vagus nerve, which may be needed if you do other things such as talking to the media, singing and running, and feeding if you have trouble swallowing.

You will need to visit your doctor daily to make sure that the pulse generator is working properly and that it has not slipped out of place. When performing any medical tests, such as magnetic resonance imaging (MRI) that may mess with your system, check with your doctor.

Evidence

Stimulation of the inserted nerve vagus is not a treatment for epilepsy. After the treatment, most people with epilepsy will not stop having seizures and completely take epilepsy medication. But many are likely to have more episodes, down to 20 to 50%. The duration of the seizure may also decrease.

Once you experience any significant reduction in epilepsy, it may take months or even a year or longer of relaxation. Stimulation of the vagus nerve may also shorten recovery time after a seizure. Patients who have had the stimulation of the vagus nerve to cure epilepsy may also experience changes in mood and quality of life.

Research on the advantages of implanted vagus nerve stimulation for depression treatment is still mixed. Several studies suggest the effects of vagus nerve stimulation for enhanced anxiety over time, and it may take at least several months before you experience any changes in your symptoms of depression. Stimulation of the embedded vagus nerve does not function for everyone and is not meant to replace conventional therapies.

Furthermore, this treatment may not be covered by some health insurance providers.

Implanted vagus nerve stimulation trials as a cure for disorders such as Alzheimer's disease, nausea, and rheumatoid arthritis were too small to draw some definitive conclusions about how well it could function for these issues. There is a need for further research.

PSYCHOPHYSIOLOGY

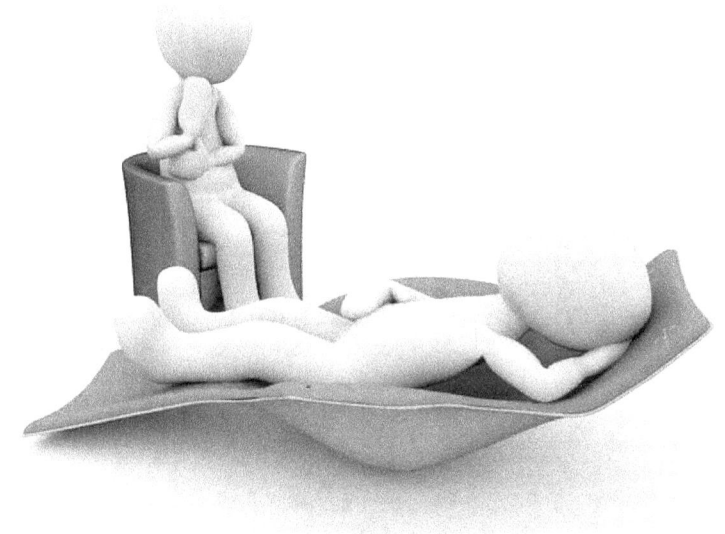

Definition

Psychophysiology is the field of psychology that deals with the relationship between psychological (psyche) and physical (physiological) processes; it is the scientific study of brain-body interaction. The

Psychophysiology area is based on the work of psychiatrists, psychologists, biochemists, neurologists, physicists, and other researchers.

Physical symptoms that are partially caused by emotional factors are characterized by a Psychophysiological condition. Some of the most prominent disease-forming emotional states are depression, stress, and terror. Migraine headaches, attention deficit hyperactivity disorder (ADHD), arthritis, ulcerative colitis, and heart disease are common psychosomatic conditions.

Origins

Historically, there has been a large gap between Psychophysiology views between the allopathic (mainstream) and traditional health cultures. While the allopathic medical field continues to follow the Cartesian health paradigm, where the mind and body are seen as distinct, the alternative medical field is firmly rooted in the idea that mind and body are intricately related. Treatment is generally aimed at repairing and treating individual conditions in the body in the mainstream medical community. Alternative health care providers are striving to look at the symptoms or cause of the underlying pathology. While the latter focuses on individual aspects of an entire system, the latter category attempts to address the whole person, mind and body, feelings, and physical symptoms. We assume mental processes influence body systems intricately, and vice versa.

The world is undergoing an ever-growing paradigm shift with a more holistic mindset in which the body and mind are no longer seen as distinct, but as intricately interrelated. Medically and socially, Western society has reached the point that integrative mind/body medicine is gradually being centered. Many clinicians and doctors choose to use treatments based on the holistic concepts of seeing psyche (mind) and some (physical body) as one or closely connected. We use modalities such as mindfulness, yoga, bodywork, and methods of imagination in attempts to alleviate general stress and heal multiple psychosomatic diseases.

Benefits

The Psychophysiology area leads the way for ongoing research into the intricacies of the interaction between mind and body. Applied Psychophysiology reports on the impact of emotional states of the central nervous system through studying and collecting information on sleep patterns, heart rate, digestive activity, immune response, and brain function. Electroencephalograms (EEGs), magnetic resonance imaging (MRI), and computerized axial tomography (CAT) scans are used to test these variables. The study of Psychophysiology was applied to many fields of alternative medicine, from psychotherapy and hypnosis to bodywork and mindfulness, in an attempt to measure the effectiveness of different therapeutic methods.

There are plenty of observations of the influence of emotional states on specific physiological processes. For example, the link between depression and heart disease and the correlation between post-traumatic stress disorder, irritable bowel syndrome, and fibromyalgia have been shown. This field hopes to improve the healing capacity of treatments by documenting the effects of emotions on health.

There are several interpretations of what might look like healthy

Psychophysiology. There are common features, however, that speak of a healthy mind/body. Eventually, if inner and cognitive consciousness is powerful enough to create a sense of identity, equilibrium, and existence in the body of a person, such a holistic state exists. The disease may be present in such a country, yet there is more combat energy to cure this fundamental systemic concept. This fact is proved by science. It has been shown that therapies that integrate mind/body processes help the healing processes for numerous diseases.

Individuals can undergo physical instability when pressures, traumas, or crippling emotional states are present. For instance, if such a sting is given to an individual with a known allergy to bee stings, the natural reaction might be panic. Blood pressure and heart rate increase as a result of this psychological response, gastrointestinal function decline, and the person becomes dizzy. If emotional stresses or traumas of this type remain in the body/mind for extended periods, an imbalance may eventually manifest in the health system, as when individuals under chronic stress succumb to disease or illness. The Psychophysiology research demonstrates that the most effective treatments are those that tackle both the emotional and physical dimensions of the disorder.

Treatments

Psychosomatic treatments from both the allopathic and alternative medical worlds are being synthesized. Methods range from medication therapy and biofeedback to meditation, yoga, and massage therapy. It has been shown that many treatments are effective; individuals have the freedom and responsibility to discover the treatments that have the most personal benefit for themselves. In one man, what is successful may not work for another. Consumers are encouraged to assess options, practitioners, and their individual needs. The field of Psychophysiology is conducting research aimed at improving consumer information.

Treatments are generally selected if they complement and enhance an individual's awareness of the relationship between body and mind. These activities are most successful by influencing the brain to influence the body in maintaining overall health problems, and vice versa. For example, meditation, a mind-centered activity, and Rolfing, a form of therapeutic bodywork, are two disciplines that have proved effective in establishing this awareness. Treatments that work with both physiology and psychology at the same time are of great benefit. This comprehensive approach can be achieved through the combination of modalities that complement each other. Sources include the integration of psychotherapy with bodywork and meditation, imagination, and yoga with certain opioid treatments.

Mind/Body

Meditation is an ancient process that has great potential to calm the mind, calm the emotions, and balance the physiology. For centuries, the art of meditation has been the focus of Eastern peoples and their traditions. Meditative techniques vary from attracting attention to the breath, chanting a mantra (a specific pre-established word or phrase), or focusing one's gaze on a specific, unchanging image (a technique of visualization). Focusing awareness on body sensations can interrupt unhealthy thinking patterns, reducing or preventing the physiological effects of stress. Studies, as well as experiential phenomena, have shown that meditation reduces blood pressure, muscle pain, and cholesterol while improving digestion, relieving anxiety and depression, improving immunity, and boosting energy levels. Ultimately, meditation can lead to the psychological and physiological knowledge of one's self. Healing is taking place out of this state of embodied presence and attention.

Body/Mind

By working through the body, some forms of bodywork have been successful in affecting the mind. Emotions, thoughts, and feelings may be in the body, just as they are in mind. For instance, the body of a depressed person can reflect the emotional state through hunched shoulders, sad facial expressions, and slow movement. Psychology has shown that a person will experience corresponding and measurable effects in mind by adopting positive physical expressions such as a smile or an improved posture. These relationships are being experimentally validated by the science of Psychophysiology.

By manipulating the body's structure during bodywork, a healer can affect both physiological and psychological health directly or indirectly. Both the new changes in physiology, as well as the changes in consciousness and awareness of physically existing patterns, provide benefits from this type of therapy. Healer and client break up old patterns in the physical tissue, mind, and emotions by becoming aware of such relationships between body and mind. Overall, freedom of body/mind is enhanced, bringing with it a greater opportunity for a holistic state of health.

Research & General Acceptance

Interest in the relationship between mind and body is as ancient as it is vast, and this connection is being researched and validated by the field of Psychophysiology. The allopathic medical world has achieved great breakthroughs in human health, particularly in the treatment of injuries and diseases that are traumatic and life-threatening. A more holistic and preventive approach to health care is being sought in medical, social, and environmental terms, one that integrates and balances the relationship between mind and body. There is a lot of work being done to develop new knowledge; the Psychophysiology field is a major contributor to the exploration.

UNDERSTANDING THE PSYCHO-EMOTIONAL ROOTS OF DISEASE

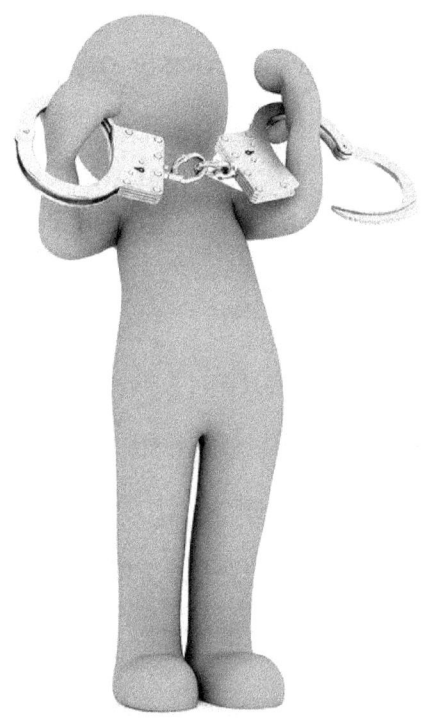

The beliefs that you hold about yourself and the world, your emotions, memories, and habits all have an impact on mental and physical health.

Healers have been thinking about the connection between mental and physical health for centuries. In recent years, science has begun to recognize the powerful connections that can directly affect health outcomes through emotional, spiritual, and behavioral factors. As research is being conducted in the field of mind-body medicine, emotions and patterns of thought can contribute to imbalances in the body, and therapies such as hypnosis, visual imaging, meditation, yoga, and biofeedback are being used to restore balance and promote health.

The beliefs that you hold about yourself and the world, emotions, memories, and habits can all have an impact on mental and physical health. The psycho-emotional roots of health and disease are these connections between what is happening in your mind and heart and what is happening in your body.

Let's take a closer look.

The connection between the mind and the body takes place both physically and chemically. The brain is the hardware that enables you to experience mental states that are labeled as the "mind." This "mind" concept includes mental states, including thoughts, beliefs, attitudes, and emotions. Different mental states can affect biological functioning positively or negatively. This is because the nervous, endocrine, and immune systems share a common chemical language that enables constant communication between mind and body through messengers such as hormones and neurotransmitters.

Neurological pathways, for example, connect parts of the brain that process emotion to the spinal cord, muscles, cardiovascular system, and digestive tract. This makes it possible to trigger physical symptoms by major life events, stresses, or emotions. You may have experienced this aspect of the connection between the mind and the body when you feel butterflies in your stomach when you feel nervous, or when you feel your heart pounding out of your chest when you are under intense stress.

These intersecting systems help to establish the connection between the mind and the body that influences health maintenance or disease development. Emotions such as anxiety, for example, can trigger increased stress hormones that can suppress the immune system and set the stage for infection or cancer development.

The Impact of Vibration

Thoughts and emotions also bring waves that influence the physiological state of biochemistry, cell, and overall. The body is made up of hydrogen and liquids at a physical level, which is in constant motion.

Science shows that thoughts, words, and feelings can change the water and cells' crystal structure, which can change their function. Positive, loving, and motivating thoughts and emotions vibrate in unison with your cells because they share a similar rhythm that helps them to function as well as possible. Indeed, one study found that the type of vibrations or patterns of energy carried by certain words and intentions can cause physical changes in the structure of DNA that affect how the genetic code is translated to make different proteins that become your body's building blocks.

This may explain why techniques such as affirmations and hypnotherapy can affect the human body with such strong effects. Sometimes, the emotions are also conveyed as words that bring these infectious impulses and then serve as repetitive patterns and activities that further affect health.

The Body Feels Emotion

Within the body, emotions such as anger, fear, guilt, anxiety, sadness, resentment, jealousy, depression, and stress can manifest and contribute to imbalance and illness. You probably already know that anxiety can contribute to gastrointestinal discomfort, for instance, or how stress can lead to headaches.

In different areas of your body, physiological sensations occur when you experience emotional states such as sadness, joy, or anger. Scientists have created maps of emotions, showing body areas that are activated when participants in the study have experienced different emotions.

This is a multi-directional connection. Emotional experiences have an impact on your body's behavior and physiology. In the other direction, your perception of these body changes triggered by emotion also affects your emotions that are consciously felt.

Stuck or repressed emotions seem to harm physical health in particular. One study showed that people who repress their emotions are more likely to disrupt the normal balance of the cortisol stress hormone compared to people who freely express their emotions. Over time, persistent psychological stress can affect how the body works on a hormonal and immunological level, leading to cancer and cardiovascular disease growth and progression. Studies show, for example, that having imbalances in how the nervous system regulates the overall response to stress, such as producing too high or too low levels of stress hormones such as cortisol and epinephrine/adrenaline, can predict early death in patients with metastatic breast cancer.

What You Believe Can Lead to Disease

Because of this connection between mind and body, the way you think and feel, and the deep-seated patterns of belief that you hold can all contribute to disease development. If you are not exploring and dealing with painful emotions, they can create an underlying sense of anxiety, depression, or anger that can physically disrupt the natural healing ability of the body.

While coping with chronic pain, one common way you can perceive the combination of perceptions and physical sensations. Essentially, pain is a combination of the physical sensations that you experience, the emotions that you feel, and the pain's meaning.

Our neural pathways share similarities to emotional suffering, physical pain, and other stimuli. For example, rage or anxiety feelings may interrupt the heart's daily pounding and the breath's steady stream. This also stimulates the sympathetic nervous system in the same way that occurs when you encounter a threat, generating an even stronger sense of discomfort and pain. This form of behavior can be seen playing out in people who lack social support, who are more likely to have heart and other health problems than those with stable and healthy relationships.

Another example of the strong connection between mind and body is that reducing depression symptoms that increase cancer survival rates. Psychological support is important in coping with feelings and shifting perceptions and can help to reduce both suicidal and inflammatory symptoms. It means that mental-body wellbeing is positively affected by emotional and social support.

Healing Mind, Body, and Spirit

This takes a combination of biological, spiritual, and emotional approaches to treat and prevent disease. There are several solutions to the mind-body that can help you process your thoughts and achieve internal and external health.

You need to remain present and mindful to prevent the development of negative emotions. Paying attention helps you to recognize and interpret feelings when they emerge and choose how you respond. Talking about them is one way to express, feel, and get your feelings out effectively. This can be done clearly when speaking to a trusted friend and therapist — or a journaling activity on paper.

Meditation is another important activity in the brain-body to become more conscious and to concentrate the mind. The regular practice of mindfulness is a particularly effective way for the brain to modulate emotional responses and the associated neurochemical changes that can otherwise fill the body with toxic stress hormones.

Certain techniques that concentrate on the body, brain, and actions communication include:
- Yoga
- Mindful breathing practices
- Tai chi
- Hypnotherapy
- Biofeedback

They can all be valuable tools to raise awareness of the biological processes of the body, such as heart rate and breathing patterns, and help you manage emotions and reduce their neurophysiological impacts.

Using these mind-body techniques will help you regain control of your psycho-emotional health and create an environment that promotes wellbeing rather than illness within the body.

HOW TO STRENGTHEN YOUR VAGUS NERVE TO UPGRADE YOUR WHOLE BODY

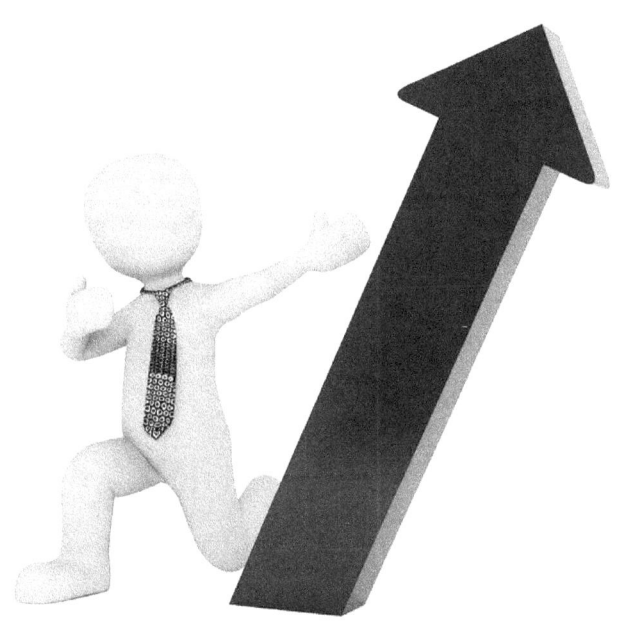

The vagus pathway is a nervous system that connects outside the brain and regulates many organs in the body — heart, lungs, gut, liver, and more.

Modern medicine treats individual organs as the disease area and ignores the fact that your brain and the nervous system tells what to do with your organs. Your bodies regularly send your brain a status check to comment on how things are going through the vagus nerve.

It's a street in two ways. When all goes well, the status quo is maintained by your brain. When an organ struggles, it may signal more resources to your brain. The vagus nerve brings the message from your brain to your organs to slow down when it's time for your body to spring into action.

Your vagus nerve needs to be in working order to ensure that nothing is lost in translation. It's up to your brain and organs to regulate things like:
- Hunger hormones
- Inflammation
- Anxiety
- The immune response

Because there's so much involved in the vagus nerves, it must work properly. Read on to find out how by vagus toning you could help the vagus nerve.

IT'S CLICHE, BUT TAKE DEEP BREATHS

There is a relationship that is modulated by the vagus nerve between respiration and heart rate. This is why the regular practice of yoga reduces overall stress.
Breathing yoga and breathing guided exercises will calm your heart rate and reduce your blood pressure. Breathing exercises increased vagal tone in an experimental group and effectively managed prehypertension.

In one study, slow breathing exercises in healthy participants improved autonomic functions. Fast breathing wasn't. That's because it makes your body think you're running from predators. This sets off the alarm bells in your body and triggers a stress response.

BOX BREATHING

If you're panicking or about to blow a gasket, try box breathing.

- Inhale for a count of four.
- Hold for a count of four.
- Exhale for a count of four.
- Wait for a count of four.
- Repeat until your hands are back on the controls.

Trace your finger in the air in a square pattern the first few times. When you're frazzled, it'll help you remember how to do it.

This gradual expanding of the lungs signals to slow down to your brain, sending a feeling of calm throughout your whole nervous system. Your vagus nerve connects all of this signaling and releases acetylcholine, a calming chemical that you can shoot at any time with relaxation techniques.

CHILL OUT, LITERALLY

Using the vagus response to the cold tones, slowing the activation of the sympathetic nervous system. Regular cold bursts significantly lower the indicators for pressure. Cold exposure helped relieve signs of depression and anxiety that the vagus nerve could modulate.

It stimulates digestion by stimulating the vagal pathways. Due to anxiety, when the metabolism of rats slowed down, cold stimulation reactivated the gastric nerves and reactivated everything.

KEEP YOUR GUT HAPPY

Have you ever heard of the axis of the gut-brain? It applies to the micro-organisms that interact with your brain in your digestive system.
Your microbiota is your body and skin's population of helpful microbes. Most often, when someone

speaks about the microbiome, they talk about your intestines and colon bacteria.

The scientific community is discovering more and more ways that the microbiota impacts the entire body as the science of the microbiome grows. Work on the link between the microbiota and mood is increasing, and contact between the intestine and the brain relies on the vagus nerve — shock.

Animal models and human studies support the idea of a thriving microbiome curbing anxiety and improving your mood. Some research looked at this effect with and without an intact vagus nerve to see if it has anything to do with vagal pathways.

Rodents that supplemented with certain strains of probiotics showed decreases in indicators of anxiety and depression, but not in animals whose vagus nerves had been cut before the experiment. Healthy women who eat four weeks of fermented food showed positive changes in brain function, particularly in those parts of the brain which regulate emotion and perception. From the animal studies and what researchers now know about the vagus nerve, you can make a solid bet that through the vagus nerve, the gut-brain interaction happens here.

A comprehensive microbiome test, such as Viome, is the best way to support your intestinal flora. Viome is a test-at-home kit for easy profiling of your microbiome, and then you get personalized dietary recommendations to get you back in balance.

Anxiety and physical illness

Anxiety— the response to "fight or flight"— can be a good thing as an ordinary feeling, encouraging us to take extra precautions. But if anxiety persists in the absence of fighting or fleeing, it can not only interfere with our daily lives but also undermine our physical health. Evidence suggests that several chronic medical conditions are at higher risk for people with anxiety disorders. These may also have more severe symptoms when they become ill and a higher risk of death.

The anatomy of anxiety

Anxiety is a stress reaction that has both physical and psychological characteristics. In the amygdala, a brain region that regulates many intense emotional responses, the feeling is thought to emerge. When neurotransmitters carry the impulse to the sympathetic nervous system, the levels of heart and breathing rise, muscles contract, and blood flow are transferred from the abdominal organs to the brain. Anxiety trains us to face a challenge in the short term by alerting the brain. But it can be harmful in its physical effects, inducing lightheadedness, vomiting, diarrhea, and frequent urination. And if it persists, our mental and physical health may be affected by anxiety.

Anxiety as an illness

Anxiety-related disease physiology research is still new, but evidence of reciprocal control between feelings and physical activity is increasing. Yet anxiety is often unidentified as a source of other disorders, such as abuse of substances or physical addiction, which may result from attempts to quench anxiety feelings. And in the various signs of chronic conditions such as irritable bowel syndrome (IBS) and migraine headaches, it is often ignored.

Approximate 40 million people with anxiety disorders, nearly two-thirds are female. What people have in common with these disorders is unwarranted fear or distress that interferes with everyday life. Anxiety frequently plays a role in the syndrome of somatic symptoms, marked by physical symptoms such as discomfort, vomiting, fatigue, and dizziness that have no clear physical cause.

Many chronic physical ailments, including heart disease, chronic respiratory illnesses, and stomach problems, also caused anxiety. When anxiety has been untreated by people with these disorders, the disease itself is harder to treat, their physical symptoms often get worse, and they die sooner in some cases.

Anxiety disorders and their symptoms

Disorder	Symptoms
Generalized anxiety disorder	Exaggerated health, security, money, and other everyday issues that last six months or more. Muscle pain, tiredness, headaches, nausea, breathlessness, and insomnia are often

	accompanied.
Phobias	Irrational fear of particular things and circumstances, such as snakes (Arachnophobia), being in crowds (Agoraphobia) or being in confined spaces (Claustrophobia).
Social anxiety disorder (social phobia)	In normal social encounters, intense self-consciousness, intensified by a feeling of being observed and judged by others and a fear of humiliation.
Post-traumaticstress	Reliving an intense physical

disorder (PTSD)	or emotional threat or injury in vivid dreams, flashbacks, or tormented memories (e.g., childhood abuse, fighting, or earthquake). Other symptoms include sleeping or concentration difficulties, angry outbursts, emotional withdrawal, and increased surprise response.
Obsessive/compulsive disorder (OCD)	Obsessive thoughts, such as an irrational fear of contamination, accompanied by compulsive acts such as repetitive hand washing to alleviate the anxiety generated by the thoughts.

Panic disorder	Recurrent bouts, followed by rapid heartbeat, vomiting, dizziness, and fatigue, with unprovoked sensations of fear and impending doom.

Anxiety and gastrointestinal disorders

Approximately 10% to 20% of Americans suffer from the two most common digestive functional disorders — IBS and functional dyspepsia (stomach upset). The nerves that control digestion seem to be hypersensitive to stimuli in these disorders. Since these conditions do not result in lesions such as ulcers or tumors, they are not considered life-threatening. But their symptoms— abdominal pain, bloating, and IBS diarrhea or constipation; and functional dyspepsia pain, nausea, and vomiting — may be chronic and hard to tolerate.

There are no concrete statistics on the prevalence of anxiety disorders in individuals with active digestive disorders, but a 2007 New Zealand study of subjects with gastroenteritis (digestive tract inflammation) found a correlation between high levels of anxiety and the incidence of IBS after infection with the intestine.

Chronic respiratory disorders and anxiety

During asthma, inflamed airways spasmodically constrict, increasing airflow through the lungs. In chronic obstructive pulmonary disease (COPD), a lack of elasticity in the lungs exacerbates the swelling of the airways: not only is it difficult for air to enter the bloodstream, but the lungs do not fill and remove oxygen.

While the results vary, most studies found a high rate of symptoms of anxiety and panic attacks in patients with chronic respiratory disease, with more risky women than men. Anxiety has been associated with more frequent hospitalization and more extreme pain at each stage of lung function in several studies involving COPD patients. So even if depression does not hinder the disease's development, the quality of life requires a substantial cost.

Anxiety and heart disease

Anxiety disorders were also associated with heart disease progression and coronary problems in people with heart disease already. In the Nurses' Health Study, women with the highest levels of phobic anxiety were 59 percent more likely than women with the lowest levels of anxiety to have a heart attack, and 31 percent more likely to die from one. In the Women's Health Initiative, data from 3,300 postmenopausal women showed that a history of full-blown panic attacks tripled the risk of a coronary event or stroke.

Two studies— one involving the Harvard Medical School and the Lown Cardiovascular Research Institute; the other involving several Canadian medical colleges— concluded that those with an anxiety disorder were twice as likely to have a heart attack as those with no history of anxiety disorders.

Physical benefits of treating anxiety

Successful therapies in the treatment of anxiety disorders can ease the symptoms of chronic gastrointestinal and respiratory diseases. These therapies can play an important role in heart disease prevention and treatment. These are the methods that are better studied: cognitive-behavioral counseling. The mental element helps people recognize and prevent anxiety-generating feelings, and the component of action helps them learn how to react differently in anxiety-provoking scenarios. Treatment specifics depend on the type of anxiety. For instance, patients with a widespread anxiety disorder or panic disorder may be asked to look into their lives for habits and patterns that foster a sense of fear. Relaxation techniques may also be taught to decrease anxiety

THE POLYVAGAL THEORY

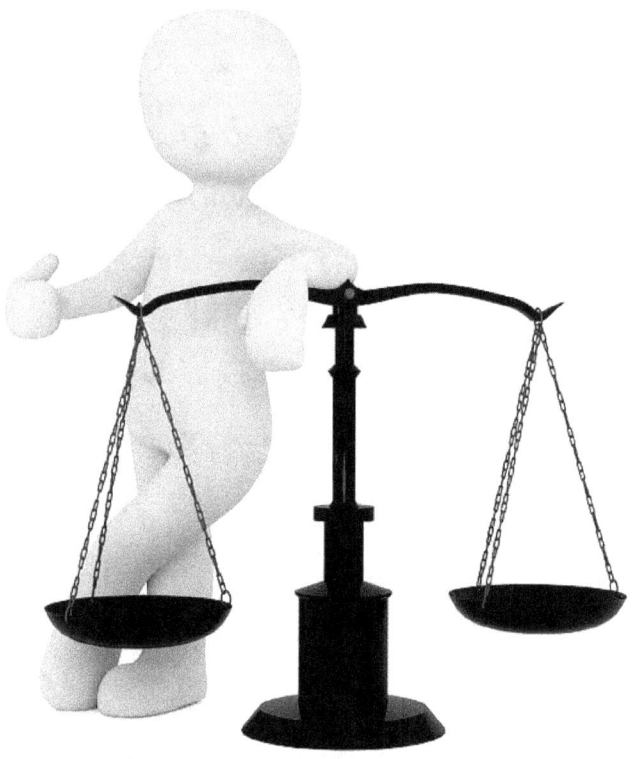

The polyvagal theory has been named' Polus,' or multiple, and the nerve running through the human body is' vagus.' It is a tool for dealing through pain and social connections based on how the nervous system responds with external stimuli ranging from security to risk. Tony Buckley, an authority on this subject, spoke to us about Polyvagal's theory and how to use it in psychology and psychotherapy.

Safety connectedness

Protection (and how the vagus nerve responds to it) is the polyvagal hypothesis. So it's all about connection because when we feel safe, we feel close to others. The theory then linked the idea of social contact as a response to a rehabilitation process from trauma.

An illusion is a term coined by Stephen Porges, the author of The Polyvagal Theory, referring to the illusion of safety and the risk we are all continuously doing without being mindful of. It is the sense of fear that tells us that someone around us is willing to cause trouble and hurt us. However, people may have a faulty sense of perception where there is no risk. It's also a response to trauma that places all the senses on high alert.

Calming the nervous system

When the alarm systems are set on high, how do we reset them? We cannot use the mind to turn it off because it's a body machine (that's why, while we're panicking, the reason doesn't work). Instead, we must use our brains.

The body is regulated by two mechanisms—the cranial nerve (controlled by our five senses) and the vagus nerve that regulates the brain, lungs, and digestive tract. Therefore, to regulate our physical reactions, we need to know how to affect our vagus nerve. So, our muscles need to be cool. This can be accomplished by grounding exercises, breathing, listening to soothing music, shaking off stress, etc. We are all special, so we're going to have to play with what fits for us.

The Window of Affective Tolerance

The sensitivity window is a perfect way to understand intense and hypo anticipation as felt in times of distress.

If we stay in' optimum arousal,' we may function normally, but if we become' hyper-aroused' to get us ready for action, we can feel anxiety instead. This condition was consistent with injury reactions to battle and flight. We can find ourselves in' hypo-arousal' at the opposite end of the spectrum, which can dull us to outside stimuli but can also lead us to shut down completely as per the flop and freeze trauma responses.

Vagus Nerve Systems

The vagus nerve covers three associated systems within the body and responds to various levels of threat.

Safety–social engagement system This collects signals from others from body language, facial expression, and voice tone and (if friendly) calms us down. This system can bypass stress hormones that are activated in us by other people.

Danger–sympathetic nervous system Increasing body blood flow and pain, dilating eyes, speeding heart rate, and respiration, and increasing blood pressure and blood pressure

Health risk–parasympathetic nervous system

is Also known as the rest or digestive process, as it will conserve energy in health-threatening situations as it decreases heart rate, raises intestinal and gland function, and relaxes gastrointestinal tract sphincter muscles. This is best seen in the opossum that so convincingly plays dead that its victims will go home, leaving it to run when the coast is clear.

The vagal irony is that if driven too far, certain devices can also destroy us if they can be shut down for safety!

Immobilization may be healthy (rest and repair) or for survival (death fired). Likewise, activation has the same two aspects of adrenalized activity (such as roller coasters) and risk practice. However, our body responds to trauma; it's positive that it does anything at all–the body does its best to keep us safe at all times.

Understanding the polyvagal system in therapy

Through counseling, using the social engagement model, we can use this understanding of the polyvagal system. Because counseling is focused on a therapeutic relationship, we can use this to help the patient heal from depression by providing a safe' other' that can be experienced and reacted to by the client's social engagement process. Once the customer feels comfortable with us, we will help them work through the pain and meet other' normal' people in their lives and extend the peace outside the counseling area.

The Vagus Nerve

The 10th cranial nerve is the vagus nerve, a fiber system that connects the throat, heart, and brain. The name derives from the Latin root vagus, meaning wandering as the nerve can communicate signals between such different parts of the body. About 80% of the vagus nerve fibers are afferent, meaning that these fibers send signals to the brain from the organs. Such afferent fibers relay sensory information about the organs ' condition (how fast the heart beats, how much you swallow, how large your pupils are). The remaining fibers are efferent, so the brain can relay and alter the function of these organs (we will discuss these fibers in the next articles more). In the nervous system, the function of the vagus nerve is to maintain a balance between the various internal organs, including the heart. This equilibrium state is called homeostasis and may be related to temperature, activation, chemistry, and other factors. This nerve is particularly important as an organ's state of equilibrium can vary with context.

For instance, if it's warm outside, your blood will circulate and disperse heat throughout your body. If it's cold outside, however, your body will keep your blood circulating through your major organs to keep it warm. The arteries in your extremities can limit blood flow to a certain degree. You may notice that in cold weather, your fingers and toes are particularly cold as they are the furthest parts of your body from your heart, and the blood does not circulate to them. You may feel frustrated that your hands are hot, but for your major organs, your body retains homeostasis in terms of temperature, so be grateful for your vagus and make sure you wear a coat and gloves.

Due to social circumstances, such as the existence of a stressor, homeostasis can also change. Of course, your heart should be relaxed and beat 60-80 times a minute. However, if a lion chases you or you're in the middle of a marathon, your heart should beat faster and pump more oxygen. Your goal is to go further in both cases so that oxygen and blood circulate to help you achieve this goal. Alternatively, when you're nervous, your heart also tends to race, like when you've got to take an important exam, or you're getting ready to talk to that particular person. In these situations, running may seem less helpful to your brain. You're not getting ready to fight and run, but as if there is a real threat, the body is displaying a stress response. The polyvagal hypothesis discusses the various types of stress responses.

The word polyvagal refers to the fact that there is a myelinated and unmyelinated branch in the vagus. Myelin sheath is the fatty layer that lines certain nerves and makes it possible to send signals faster and more accurately. The unmyelinated branch is more primitive, lacking this myelination, and consequently, it is also less quick and organized than the myelinated branch. The myelinated version can be pictured as a highway with stoplights — the road is asphalt, and you can drive fast, but the street is still designed, and drivers can travel safely. The branch that is unmyelinated is more like a bumpy dirt road. It's not perfectly paved, but fast driving is difficult. It is also not monitored so that it may be a bit haphazard, and you may run the risk of an accident.

Such divisions, including the heart, establish homeostasis between various internal organs. Via three different stages of neuronal regulation, they can do this. Such levels are the unmyelinated vagus, the sympathetic-adrenal process, and the myelinated vagus, for the least to the most advanced.

Anatomical Terminology

The terms used by anatomists and health care providers can be confusing to the uninitiated. The purpose of this language, however, is not to confuse but to increase accuracy and reduce medical errors. For example, is a scar "above the wrist" two or three inches from the hand on the forearm? Or is it at the hand's base? Is it on the front of the hand or back? We eliminate ambiguity by using precise anatomical terminology. Anatomical terms originate from the vocabulary of ancient Greek and Latin. Because these languages are no longer used in daily conversation, there is no change in the meaning of their words.

Roots, prefixes, and suffixes are biological words. A term's root sometimes refers to an organ, tissue, or disease, while the root is often represented by the prefix or suffix. The prefix "hyper-" means "high" or "over" in the hypertension disorder, for example, and the root word "tension" refers to pressure, so the word "hypertension" refers to abnormally high blood pressure.

Anatomical Position

Anatomists standardize the way they view the body to further improve accuracy. Just as maps are normally oriented at the top with the north, the standard body "map" or anatomical position is that of the body standing upright, with the feet of the width of the shoulder and parallel toes forward.

Confusion is minimized by using this standard position. No matter how the descriptive body is oriented, the terms are used as if they are in an anatomical position. For instance, there would be a scar on the palm side of the wrist in the "anterior (front) carpal (wrist) region." Even if the hand were palm down on a table, the word "anterior" would be used.

A lying body is either described as prone or supine. Prone describes a face-down orientation, and a face-up orientation is described by supine. These terms are sometimes used during specific physical examinations or surgical procedures to describe the body's position.

Regional Terms

The various areas of the human body have specific terms to help increase precision. Note that the term "brachium" or "arm" is reserved for the "upper arm" and "ante brachium" or "forearm" is used instead of the term "lower arm." Similarly, "femur" or "thigh" is correct, and "leg" or "crus" is reserved for the lower limb portion between the knee and ankle.

Directional Terms

To define the relative positions of different body components, these words are important. For example, an anatomist could describe one tissue band as "inferior to" another or a doctor could describe a tumor as "superficial to" a deeper body structure. Commit these words in memory to avoid misunderstanding when you research and explain the positions of different parts of the body.

- Front (or ventral) Describes the front or the front of the body — the toes in front of the foot.
- Back (or dorsal) Describes the back and line to the rear of the head. The popliteus leads the patella.
- Superior (or cranial) defines a position above or above the proper body portion. The orbits are better than oris.
- Inferior (or caudal) defines a position beneath or below that of another proper part of the body, above or to the tail (in mammals,

coccyx, or lower spinal column). The pelvis is less than the uterus.
- The side or direction to the side of the body is defined laterally. The thumb (pollex) to the digits is lateral.
- Medial defines the origin and orientation of the body towards the heart. The hallux is the toe of the medium.
- Proximal defines the location of the limb closest to the body's attachment point or trunk. The brachium comes similar to the ante brachium.
- Distal defines a location in a limb that is further away from the body's attachment point or trunk. The cru to the femur is distal.
- Superficial defines a location that is near the body layer. The bones have superficial skin.
- Deeply defines a position far back from the body's bottom. The nucleus in the head is deep.

Body Planes

A section is a two-dimensional surface that has been cut into a three-dimensional structure. Modern medical imaging devices allow obtaining "virtual sections" of living bodies for clinicians. We're naming the scans. Furthermore, body parts and scans can be viewed accurately only if the audience knows the plane the segment was rendered along. A plane is a two-dimensional imaginary surface passing through the body. For physiology and surgery, three planes are commonly referred to.

- The sagittal plane is the plane that vertically divides the body or organ into the right and left sides. If this vertical plane runs down the middle of the skin, the midsagittal or median plane is called. It is called a parasagittal plane, or less commonly a longitudinal section if it divides the body into unequal right and left sides.

- The frontal plane is the line that separates the body and organ into the front portion of the body and the back portion of the body — also referred to as a coronal plane, the frontal plane.
- The transverse plane is the plane which horizontally divides the body or organ into the upper and lower portions. Transverse planes are generating images called cross-sections.

Body Cavities and Serous Membranes

By membranes, sheaths, and other mechanisms dividing compartments, the body retains its internal organization. The largest body compartments are the dorsal (posterior) cavity and the ventral (anterior) cavity. Such cavities house and defend fragile internal organs, and as they conduct their functions, the ventral cavity makes significant changes in the size and shape of the organs. For example, the lungs, chest, stomach, and intestines may expand and contract without distorting other tissues or interfering with surrounding organ function.

Subdivisions of the Posterior (Dorsal) and Anterior (Ventral) Cavities

The cavities posterior (dorsal) and anterior (ventral) are subdivided into smaller cavities. The cranial cavity houses the brain in the posterior (dorsal) cavity, and the spinal cavity (or vertebral cavity) contains the spinal cord. Just as a single, unified structure is created by the brain and spinal cord, so are the cranial and spinal cavities which contain them. The brain and spinal cord are covered by the skull and vertebral column bones and cerebrospinal fluid, a blood-produced colorless fluid that cushions the brain and spinal cord in the posterior (dorsal) cavity.

The two major subdivisions of the anterior (ventral) cavity are the thoracic cavity and the abdominopelvic cavity. The thoracic cavity is the anterior cavity's upper segment and is surrounded by the rib cage. The thoracic cavity comprises the mediastinum's lungs and heart. The diaphragm covers the thoracic cavity's surface and separates it from the upper abdominopelvic cavity. The most important cavity in the body is the abdominopelvic cavity. Although the abdominopelvic space is not separated by any membrane, it may be useful to distinguish between the abdominal cavity, the division housing the digestive organs, and the pelvic cavity, the division hosting the reproductive organs.

WHY VAGAL TONE MATTERS

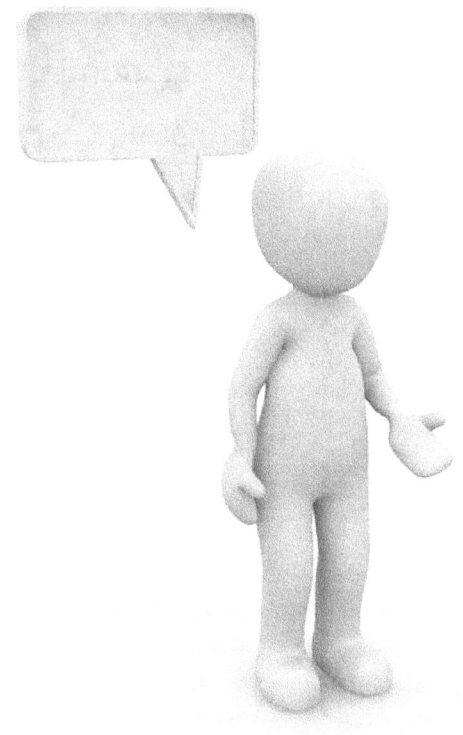

Essentially, Vagal tone is how good and "sound" the nerve of the Vagus is. The higher the vagal tone, the easier it is to get into a state of relaxation.

Research published in 2013 in Psychological Science reveals a positive feedback loop between high vagal tone, good physical health, and good emotional health. While the researchers agree that "the processes underlying the relationship between positive emotions and physical health remain a mystery," they identified a link between a toned Vagal nerve and better physical and emotional health. The reverse is true, as well. The better the physical and emotional health, the higher the sound of your Vagal.

What does the body's vagus nerve do?

In optimal health, the vagus nerve is an important player, particularly when entering a parasympathetic or comfortable state. Here are some of the reasons the body is affected by the Vagus nerve.

Connects the Brain to the Gut

If you've ever had a gut sensation about something, it's due to your vagus nerve. The vagus nerve links the brain to the intestine and sends information back and forth. This is also called the axis of the intestinal brain. Your gut tells details about your brain by electrical impulses called "potentials of action."

Connects the Brain to Other Organs

The vagus nerve also connects the brain with other vital organs as it passes to the intestine. This takes sensory information to the brain from the liver.

When regulating the heart rate, the vagus nerve plays an important role. The neurotransmitter acetylcholine is activated by the vagus nerve, which decreases the heart rate. The improvement in cardiac levels includes vagus nerve stimulation suppression (which ensures no release of acetylcholine). Physicians will monitor your heart rate variability (HRV) and figure out a lot about your heart and vagus nerve's wellbeing. If your HRV is low, there's a high vagal tone.

The vagus nerve also plays a role in the operation of the heart. Often responsible for telling the lungs to breathe is the acetylcholine that the vagus nerve induces to release.

Controls the Parasympathetic Nervous System

The parasympathetic nervous system is the nervous system's "stop and eats" component (as opposed to the sympathetic nervous system's fight or flight mechanism). As described above, the vagus nerve activates the release of acetylcholine (in relaxation) to suppress heart rate. The vagus nerve also plays an important role in calming and regeneration stimulation.

Stimulates Digestive Tract

It is the vagus nerve, which activates digestion. Even before eating any food, it does this. To start producing gastric juices to prepare for digestion, it sends signals to the gastrointestinal (GI) tract. If the vagus nerve is not optimal, it is not optimal for digestion.

Stimulates Memory Making

Research by the University of Virginia showed that activation of the vagus nerve could help to solidify memories by inducing norepinephrine release. In those with memory problems or those with Alzheimer's disease, this can be significant.

Prevents Chronic Inflammation

One of the vagus nerve's most remarkable features is that it can stop inflammation. In many modern diseases, from cancer to heart disease, chronic inflammation is involved. According to a Molecular Medicine study, when the vagus nerve detects inflammation (for instance, by the existence of pro-inflammatory cytokine), it activates the production of anti-inflammatory neurotransmitters to control the immune system.

However, a 2016 study found that activation of the vagus nerve helped to reduce signs of rheumatoid arthritis, a condition without a cure.

Natural Ways to Stimulate the Vagus Nerve

Stimulation of the vagus nerve is necessary for optimum health. There is a system approved by the FDA that can be inserted in the skin. To activate the vagus nerve, it emits electrical impulses. However, without surgery, appliances, or side effects, there are other ways to activate the vagus nerve.

Cold therapy

Cold therapy has many benefits from faster recovery from exercise and improved immune function. Acute cold exposure, according to a 2001 report, also stimulates the vagus nerve and cholinergic neurons and nitrergic neurons through vagus nerve pathways. This means that cold exposure can also increase parasympathetic function through the nerve of the vagus, suppressing the sympathetic response (fighting and flight).

Deep Breathing

Deep, slow breathing can help induce relaxation; it is well-known. Vagal stimulation, as mentioned earlier, can cause relaxation, but the opposite is true as well. Relaxation may stimulate the nerve of the vagus. So inducing deep breathing, relaxation can help improve vagal tone. In the future, this will make it easier to enter a relaxed state!

Singing, Humming, Gargling

Singing or humming on their own may be soothing, but there is a physiological reason for it. The vocal cords are attached to the vagus nerve. Research published in Psychology's Frontiers reveals that it can be triggered by chanting, humming, and even gargling. Chewing also increases the operation of the vagus nerve (and the parasympathetic process which controls digestion, making sense!). While it may have its downsides, it means chewing gum often activates the vagus nerve.

Intermittent fasting

Intermittent fasting can enhance mental and mitochondrial function. It can also improve metabolism and reduce heart disease and cancer risk.

But it turns out that these health benefits can be correlated with the ability of intermittent fasting to activate the vagus nerve and enhance the vagal tone. A 2003 study found fasting to be a vagus nerve biochemical activator.

Wave Vibration

The scientific community has studied wave vibration heavily for its health benefits. This treatment involves sitting on a low-level vibration oscillating surface. Then these vibrations create positive stress throughout the body (like the type of stress that exercise creates). This stress, among other parts of the body, activates the vagal nerve.

Probiotics

Probiotics are an important part of the diet and benefit from digestive problems and skin problems for many illnesses. Probiotics can also be useful in stimulating the vagus nerve, and it turns out. Results from a 2011 study found that giving Lactobacillus Rhamnosus mice increased their development of GABA and decreased stress, as well as activity related to depression and anxiety.

Ironically, those who had not had a vagus nerve in the probiotics (it was removed) did not see the same effects. This suggests that there was something to do with the activation of the vagus nerve to improve stress resilience.

Healthy Fats and Omega-3s

A study published in Frontiers in Psychology in 2011 found that high fish intake was associated with a primarily parasympathetic (relaxed) nervous system and decreased vagal activity. Scientists speculated that the explanation for this was the fish's omega-3 quality.

Exercise

In a healthy lifestyle, exercising is an important part. But it seems that stimulating the vagus nerve may also be beneficial. This may be the explanation of why we can cope with exercise. One study in 2010 found that mild exercise stimulated gastric emptying and enhanced digestion. They figured out this was due to vagal stimulation.

Massage

Research suggests that in relaxing the vagus nerve, acupuncture can be helpful. There was a greater weight gain attributed to vagal operation in one 2012 study of premature infants who were massaged. We're trying to use a range of massage techniques and tools at home this is one factor.

Foot reflexology can also improve the sound of the vagus. Foot reflexology improved vagal stimulation, reduced sympathetic regulation, and lowered blood pressure, according to a study published in Alternative Therapies for Health and Medicine.

Laughter and Social Enjoyment

We all know that a good way to relax is to smile and be around friends and family. But a report in 2013 stumbled upon an interesting finding: there is a connection between mental health and social enjoyment of physical health. Positive social experiences affect positive emotions which enhance the sound of the vagus. It enhanced physical health afterward.

The study concluded that in a self-sustaining upward-spiral environment, "positive emotions, positive social interactions, and physical health impact each other." The study also found that regular meditation and constructive reinforcement can bring people into this upward spiral.

Acupuncture

The use of acupuncture by ancient Chinese medicine may be useful to activate the vagus nerve. Research shows that ear acupuncture can benefit from the following:

- heart regulation
- respiratory regulation
- gastrointestinal tract regulation

Additionally, according to a 2012 report, foot reflexology can reduce blood pressure by modulating the vagus nerve.

AN INTRODUCTION TO THE NERVOUS SYSTEM

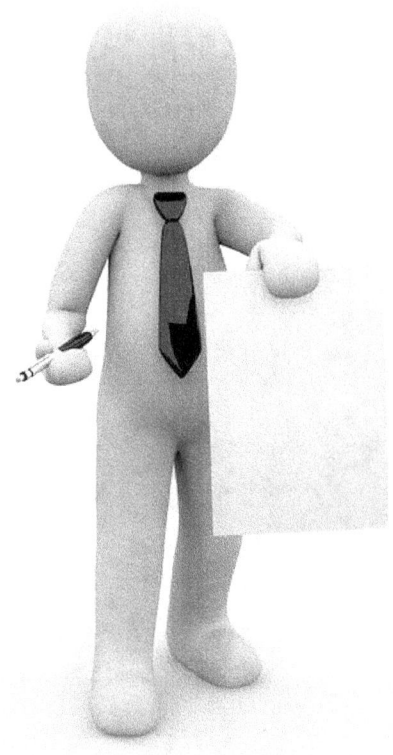

The nervous system is a specific center of organism management. It is thanks to the proper functioning of the nervous system that we are able to think, feel or perform various activities. The nervous system can be divided differently: into the central and peripheral nervous system or the somatic and autonomic nervous system. The structure of the nervous system is as complicated as its functions.

What is part of the nervous system, what are its functions and what are the diseases of the nervous system?

The nervous system is considered the most important of the systems existing in the human body. This treatment of this part of the body is caused by the fact that it is the nervous system that controls the activity of other body systems. The complexity of the structure of the nervous system is certainly not surprising - this structure performs so many functions that its complex organization basically seems understandable.

Nervous system: development
The nervous system begins to develop early - its first embryos appear in the body around the third

week of fetal life (about 18-19 days after fertilization).

The first structure of the nervous system - the neural plaque - arises from the neuroectoderm (cells of one of the three leaves of the embryo - ectoderm differentiate in it).

The next stage in the development of the human nervous system is the formation of a neural gutter, and when - around 20-25 days after fertilization - its edges become overgrown, then the neural tube develops.

During the second month of fetal life, the fetal nervous system undergoes subsequent changes. Brain bubbles are formed from the neural tube, which initiates the development of three major parts of the brain - they are:

- forebrain
- midbrain
- hindbrain

At the same time, the structures of the ventricular system of the brain are formed.

The next month of the fetus's life is the time during which blood vessels supplying CNS tissues intensively form.

In turn, the fourth month after fertilization is the time when the process of cerebral gyrification is initiated, consisting in the formation of furrows and bends within the brain.

The most important processes regarding the development of the nervous system occur during intrauterine life, but this is not synonymous with the fact that when a person comes into the world, his nervous system is fully developed.

Processes such as myelination (i.e. the formation of myelin sheaths around nerve fibers) are initiated in the womb, but they last for many long years after birth. It turns out that myelination processes can take place up to the age of 20, and sometimes even longer.

Nervous system: morphological division

The basic division of the nervous system distinguishes two parts: the central nervous system and the peripheral nervous system. The central nervous system (CNS) is an important structure of the human nervous system. This is where all the important centers responsible for controlling various body functions are located. The CNS structures include:

Located in the skull of the brain (the elements of which include the dermis, interbrain and the brainstem, which include the midbrain, bridge and medulla oblongata).

Spinal cord protected by spinal structures

CNS tissues consist of two elements. They are gray matter (made up mainly of nerve cell bodies) and white matter (consisting of fibers of cells of the nervous system).

The central nervous system is indeed the center of command of body functions, but this structure could not play its role without the peripheral nervous system - it is this second portion of the nervous system that is responsible for delivering nerve impulses from all body structures to the CNS. The peripheral nervous system includes:
- cranial nerves (of which 12 pairs are distinguished)
- spinal nerves (of which there are 31 pairs)
- nerve ganglia (located in different places of the body clusters of nerve cell bodies)
- peripheral nerve endings

Neurodegenerative diseases: causes, types, symptoms, treatment

Cerebellar tumors: causes, symptoms, treatment

Nervous system tuberculosis: causes, symptoms, treatment

Nervous system: functional division

The human nervous system can be divided not only because of its structure but also taking into account its function. In the functional division, the somatic nervous system and the autonomic nervous system are distinguished.

The somatic system is the portion of the nervous system that is primarily associated with the activities we realize. This element of the nervous system is responsible, among others for movement - these phenomena are controlled by pyramid system - is primarily involved in performing intentional and planned activities extrapyramidal system.

The somatic nervous system also receives various sensory stimuli, such as touch or temperature; it is also a structure that receives impulses from the sense organs, i.e. visual, auditory, and olfactory or taste stimuli.

The second functional element of the nervous system is the autonomic (vegetative) nervous system. The name of this element of the nervous system comes from the fact that its activity takes place completely without our conscious control. Within the autonomous system, two parts that operate in opposition to each other are distinguished:

- sympathetic nervous system
- parasympathetic system

The autonomous system is responsible for a number of different phenomena, including it affects heart function, regulates digestive system function, controls the state of the sphincter (e.g. bladder sphincter), and is also responsible for the state of the pupil (it is the autonomic system that leads to narrowing or dilatation of the pupil) and affects the condition of the respiratory tract (this system can lead to bronchoconstriction or enlargement).

Nervous system: cell structure

The basic cells that build the nervous system are neurons. There are several elements important for the functioning of the nervous system. The body of the nerve cell has two types of protrusions: shorter dendrites and longer axons.

Dendrites are primarily used to transfer information between closely located nerve cells. Axons, in turn, are definitely longer projections (in man, the length of the axon can reach up to about one hundred centimeters) and their function is to send nerve impulses over much further distances.

There may be as many as 15 billion neurons in the human nervous system, definitely - because even up to ten times more there may be other cells in it, called glial cells. These types of cells of the nervous system include, among others:

- microglia cells
- oligodendrocytes
- astrocytes
- ependemocyty

Schwann cells

Each of these types of glial cells has an important function in the nervous system. The cells involved in the formation of myelin sheaths are oligodendrocytes and Schwann cells.

Astrocytes fulfill the function of supporting neurons and have an impact on the transmission of nerve impulses, ependemocytes, in turn, are important for the proper function of the blood-brain barrier.

On the other hand, microglia cells are designed to defend the structures of the nervous system - the term microglia is defined as specific cells of the nervous system of the immune system.

HOW DOES IT WORK

The nervous system includes all nerve cells of the human body. He communicates with the environment and at the same time manages a variety of internal mechanisms. The nervous system absorbs sensory stimuli, processes them and triggers reactions such as muscle movements or pain sensations. For example, when someone reaches for a hot stove, he or she reflexively pulls his hand back, and the nerves simultaneously send a pain signal to the brain. Metabolic processes are also controlled by the nervous system.

The nervous system contains many billions of nerve cells called neurons. Inside the brain, there are about 100 billion nerves. Every single nerve cell consists of one body and different processes. The shorter processes (dendrites) act like antennas: via them, the cell body receives signals, for example from other nerve cells. Over the long extension (axon), which can be over a meter long, the signals are forwarded.

According to the location of the nerve tracts in the body, a distinction is made between a central and a peripheral nervous system. The central nervous system (CNS) includes neural pathways in the brain and spinal cord. It is safely embedded in the skull and spinal canal in the spine. The peripheral nervous system (PNS) includes all other nerve tracts of the body.

Regardless of the situation, one speaks of an arbitrary and involuntary nervous system. The voluntary nervous system (somatic nervous system) controls all processes that are conscious and that you can influence at will. These are, for example, targeted movements of arms, legs and other body parts.

The autonomic nervous system regulates the processes in the body that cannot be controlled by the will. It is constantly active and regulates, for example, breathing, heartbeat and metabolism. It receives signals from the brain and sends them to the body. In the opposite direction, the autonomic nervous system transmits messages from the body to the brain, such as how full the bladder is or how fast the heartbeats. The autonomic nervous system can very quickly adapt to the function of the body to other conditions. For example, if a person is warm, the system increases blood flow and sweating to cool the body.

The central and peripheral nervous systems contain arbitrary and involuntary proportions. In the central nervous system, however, the two parts are strongly intertwined, while they are usually separated in other areas of the body.

The autonomic involuntary nervous system is divided into three areas:

- The sympathetic nervous system
- The parasympathetic nervous system
- The intestinal nervous system (enteric nervous system)

The sympathetic and parasympathetic nervous system (sympathetic and parasympathetic) act in the body usually as an opponent: The sympathetic prepares the organism for physical and mental performance. It ensures that the heart beats faster and stronger, expands the respiratory tract so that you can breathe better and inhibits the intestinal activity.

The parasympathetic nervous system takes care of the body's functions at rest: It activates digestion, stimulates various metabolic processes and provides relaxation. The sympathetic and parasympathetic nervous system are not always opposite; For some functions, the two systems complement each other.

The enteric nervous system describes its own nervous system of the intestine, which largely independently regulates the movement of the intestine during digestion.

We will start with a microscopic description of what makes up the nervous tissue to understand the nervous system. Then we will discuss the various macroscopic classes.

Microscopic Description:

There are two cell types that make up the body's nervous tissue: nerves and glia. Neurons are cells that process information. They communicate with each other with the use of electrical and chemical means. Electrical interaction is accomplished in the nervous system by "potentials of action." At the "synapse," which is the region where the two separate neurons interact with each other, the potential of action is transformed into a chemical signal.

Glia, on the other hand, is the cells that sustain it. There are many different types of glia, each having different functions. For example, glia known as oligodendrocytes helps isolate neuronal axons to ensure fast and efficient electrical communication in the brain and spinal cord. Another type of glia, astrocytes, is responsible for the blood-brain barrier. They also maintain the integrity of the neuron-specific chemical environment. Another type of glia, ependymal cells, ventricles column, and brain cavities filled with fluid. It is important to realize that with important functions, there are other forms of glia.

When we combine many millions of neurons and glia into structural units, we come to the basis for the macroscopic level definition of the nervous system.

Depending on anatomical location, the nervous system is usually divided into two separate divisions. Peripheral nervous system (PNS) and the central nervous system (CNS) are the divisions.

The nervous system is a complex chain of nerves and cells that carry messages from and to different parts of the body from the brain and spinal cord.
Both the central nervous system and the peripheral nervous system are part of the nervous system. The central nervous system consists of the cerebral and spinal cord, and the Somatic and Autonomic nervous systems form the peripheral nervous system.
The Central Nervous System (CNS)
There are two main components of the central nervous system: the heart and the spinal cord.

The brain is located inside the skull, shaped like a mushroom. The brain is made up of four primary parts:

- the brain stems
- the cerebrum
- the cerebellum
- the diencephalon

The weight of the brain is 1.3 to 1.4 kg. It has nerve cells called neurons, and it is called the glia that supports cells.

The brain contains two kinds of matter: gray matter and white matter. Gray matter is gaining momentum and stores it. Neuron and neuralgia cell bodies are in the gray matter. In mind, white matter holds signals from and to gray matter. It is made up of nerve fibers (axons).

The brain stem is also known as the oblongata of the Medulla. It is between the pans and the cord of the spinal cord and is only around one inch long.

The cerebrum is the major component of the brain and is carried on the brain stem. There are two hemispheres in the cerebrum. Each hemisphere controls the side of the body's activities opposite the hemisphere.

When separating the hemispheres into four lobes:
- Frontal lobe
- Temporal lobes
- Parietal lobe
- Occipital lobe

The Cerebellum

It is behind the cerebrum and below it. Also known as the forebrain stem is the Diencephalon. The thalamus and hypothalamus are included. The thalamus is where visual signals coalesce with other impulses. A smaller part of the diencephalon in the hypothalamus.

Other Parts of the Brain

Certain parts of the brain include the midbrain and the Pons:

- the midbrain includes conduction paths to and from higher and lower centers
- the pones function as a conduit to higher structures; it comprises conduction routes between the medulla and higher brain centers.

The Spinal Cord

The spinal cord is like a chain that extends from the brain along the tube. A sequence of 31 segments consists of the spinal cord. From each segment comes a pair of spinal nerves. The spinal cord area that originates from a pair of spinal nerves is called the spinal section. In the spinal cord are both motor and auditory nerves.

The spinal cord in adult women is about 43 cm long and in adult men is about 45 cm long and about 35-40 grams weighs. It is the collection of bones (backbone) within the vertebral column.

The meninges are three plates of membranes that protect both the brain and the spinal cord. The dura mater is the outermost surface. The arachnoid is the central layer, and the pia mater is the innermost layer. The meninges provide brain and spinal cord defense by serving as a foil for bacteria and other micro-organisms.

Flow of the cerebrospinal fluid (CSF) around the brain and spinal cord. The brain and spinal cord are secured and nourished.

Neurons

The neuron is the nervous system's basic unit. It is a specialized cell of conductors that receives electrochemical nerve impulses and transmits them. The neuron has a cell body and long arms that carry impulses from one part of the body to another.

The neuron has three different parts:
- the cell bodies
- dendrites
- axon

Cell Body of a Neuron

The cell body is like any other nucleus or control center cell.

Dendrites

There are several strongly branched, dense branches in the cell body that act as cables and are called dendrites. The exception is a sensory neuron that instead of many dendrites has a single, long dendrite. There are multiple thick dendrites in the motor neurons. The role of the dendrite is to carry a nerve impulse into the body of the cell.

Axon

This is a long, thin process that carries impulses to another neuron or tissue away from the cell body. Typically, there is only one axon per neuron.

Myelin Sheath

The neuron is covered by the cells of the Myelin Sheath or Schwann. These are white segmented, containing more peripheral nerves between axons and dendrites. Except at the termination point and Ranvier nodes, the covering is continuous along the axons or dendrites.

The neurilemma is the nucleus layer of Schwann cells. Its function is to regenerate damaged nerves. Nerves in the brain and spinal cord have no neurilemma and are therefore unable to recover if damaged.

Types of Neuron

The body's neurons can be categorized by structure and function. Multipolar neurons, bipolar neurons, or unipolar neurons may be multipolar neurons according to structure:

The Multipolar neurons have one axon and several dendrites.
The Bipolar neurons have one axon and one dendrite, which are normal in the brain and spinal cord. These are seen in the eye retina, the inner ear, and the (small) area of the olfactory.

One cycle of unipolar neurons spread from the cell head. The one phase is separated, with one part serving as an axon and the other as a dendrite. In the spinal cord, these are used.

The Peripheral Nervous System
There are two parts of the peripheral nervous system:

- Somatic nervous system
- Autonomous nervous system.

The Somatic Nervous System

The somatic nervous system is made up of peripheral nerve fibers that absorb sensory information and stimuli from peripheral and remote organs (those like limbs far from the brain) and take them to the central nervous system.

These are also made up of motor nerve fibers that come out of the brain and carry signals to the skeletal muscles for movement and motion. For example, the tactile nerves carry information about the temperature to the brain when approaching a warm surface, which, in effect, through the motor nerves, signals the hand's muscles to withdraw it immediately.

It takes less than a second to occur in the entire process. The neuron's cell body, which holds the information, frequently lies within the brain or spinal cord and directly projections to a skeletal muscle.

Autonomic Nervous System

The Autonomic Nervous System is another part of the nervous system. It has three parts:

- The sympathetic nervous system
- The parasympathetic nervous system
- The enteric nervous system

This nervous system regulates the muscles of the body's internal organs that are not actively controlled by people. This includes heartbeat, digestion, respiration (except breathing consciously), etc.

The autonomic nervous system's nerves enervate (internal organs) and glands' smooth unconscious muscles and allow them to act and secrete their metabolites, etc.

The third autonomic part of the nervous system is the enteric nervous system. It is also the complex network of nerve fibers inside the abdomen, such as the gastrointestinal tract, pancreas, gall bladder, etc. It has almost 100 million nerves.

Neurons in the Peripheral Nervous System

The nervous system's biggest function is the amygdale. There is one preganglionic neuron for each chain of impulses, and one in front of the cell body or ganglion, which is like a central controlling body of multiple peripheral neurons.

The preganglionic cell is either in the cortex or the tissue of the spinal cord. This preganglionic neuron projects into an autonomic ganglion in the autonomic nervous system. Afterward, the postganglionic neuron contributes to the target body.

There is only one neuron in the somatic nervous system between the central nervous system and the target body, while two nerves are used by the autonomic nervous system.

Functions of The Nervous System

The nervous system consists of two parts that are integrally joined with each other. The brain and nervous system have multiple functions that are essential for the normal functioning of the fuselage.

Gearbox of the impulse

The nerve impulse is essentially an electrical stimulus that moves over the cell membrane. It crosses axons and dendrites of neurons. It moves through the dendrites of the skin and then reaches the cell body, the axon, the axon terminals and the neuron synapse.

The synapse is a junction between two neurons where the impulse moves from one to the other. At the synapse neurotransmitters are present. It is the chemical emitters of the messengers that transmit the impulse. They include acetylcholine and norepinephrine.

The impulse connects to the next dendrite, in a chain reaction until it reaches the brain that consecutively requires the skeletal muscles to function.

The reflex arc

These reflexes are automatic and involuntary reactions. They may or may not concern the brain for example flashing does not affect the brain. The reflex arc is the main functional elements of the nervous system that helps a person respond to a stimulus.

Operations of different parts of the nervous system

The different parts of the nervous system have different functions. They can be given as follows.

Brain functions

The brain consists of several pieces. Every part has a major function:
The Cerebral cortex
Thought, voluntary movement, reasoning and perception are the main functions of the cerebral cortex.
The cortex means literally "barks" (of a tree) in Latin and is so named because it is a sheet of tissue that connects the brain outer part.

The cerebral thickness is between 3 to 7 millimeters. The right and left parts of the cerebral cortex are joined by a thick band of nerve fibers called the corpus callosum.

The cortex has many incisions and jolts to increase its surface. A jolt or protrusion on the cortex is called a gyrus (the plural of the word gyrus is "gyrus") and an incision is called a sulcature (the plural of the word sulcature is "sulcatures").

Cerebellum

The main functions of the cerebellum are maintenance of movement, rest and position. The word "cerebellum" was derived from the Latin word for "tiny brain". It is divided into two parts and has a cortex that covers the hemispheres.

Hypothalamus

The hypothalamus regulates body temperatures, emotions and hunger, thirst and controls circadian rhythms.
This dimension organ by anchor nozzle is at the controls of body temperature. It acts as a "thermostat" by detecting changes in body temperature and sends signs of adjusting the temperature.

Oblongata of brainstem or medulla

This place is essential for the duration as it regulates breathing, heart rate and blood pressure. The brainstem includes medulla, bridge, tectum, reticular formation and tegmentum.

Thalamus

Works by integrating sensory information and engine information. The thalamus receives sensory information and retransmits this detail to the cerebral cortex.

The cerebral cortex also passes information to the thalamus which then transmits this information to other regions of the brain and spinal cord.

Limbic system

This part of the brain includes the amygdala, the hippocampus, the hulled fuselages and the cingulated gyrus. These help by regulating the emotional reaction. The hippocampus is also important for learning.

Central gray nuclei

This part works in the rest and update movements. It includes structures such as Globus pallidus, caudate nucleus, subthalamic nucleus, putamen and substantia nigra.

Midbrain

This part of the brain has sites adjusting the visibility, hearing, eye movement and general fuselage movement. The structures that are components of the midbrain are upper and lower colliculi and red nucleus.

Functioning of the cerebrospinal nervous system

This system has twelve pairs of cranial nerves. These are connected to the brain and have specific functions. Each cranial nerve leaves the skull through an opening at its base.
The nerves and their functioning include:
- Olfactory - for the smell
- Optics - view
- Oculomotor - movement of eyeball, lens, and pupils
- Trochlear - movement of the upper oblique muscle of the eye
- Rigeminal - innervates the eyes, cheeks and maxillary places and chewing controls
- Abducens - movements the eye outwards

Facial - control muscles of the face, scalp, and ears; rule salivary glands; receives the sensation of taste from the previous two-thirds of the tongue
Acoustics - hearing and maintaining balance

- Glossopharyngeal - sensation of back taste of the tongue and throat
- Vagus - innervates the chest and abdominal organs
- the Spinal accessory - main movement and shoulders
- Hypoglossus - tongue control muscles

Operations of the autonomic nervous system

The autonomic nervous system is divided into benevolent and parasympathetic nervous systems. These two systems have opposite functions on the same organ sets.

The sympathetic nervous system is important during an emergency and is connected with the "fight or flight reaction". Energy is directed from digestion, there is dilation of pupils, increased heart rate, increased perspiration and salivation, etc. increased breathing.

The parasympathetic nervous system is linked with a relaxed condition. The pupils contract, energy is diverted for the digestion of food, heart rate slows down, etc.

VAGUS NERVE DYSFUNCTIONS AND ASSOCIATED DISEASES

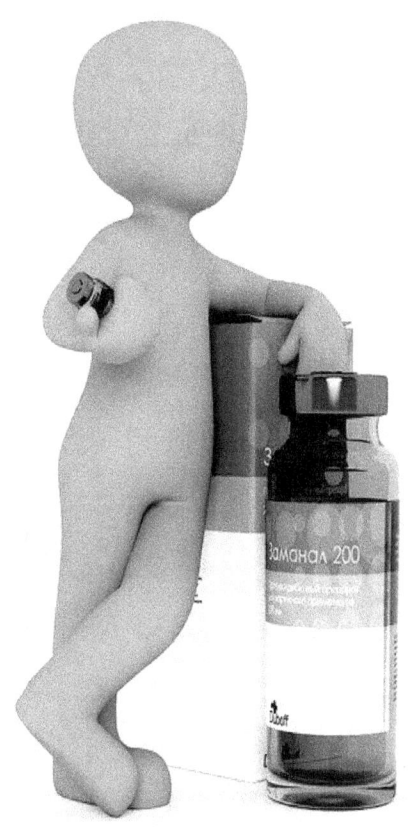

The vagus nerve is so-called because it "wanders" like a vagabond, sending to your visceral organs sensory fibers from your brainstem. The vagus nerve, the largest of the cranial nerves, regulates the parasympathetic nervous system of your internal nerve center. And it supervises a wide range of crucial functions, communicating motor and sensory impulses to each organ in the body system. A study has revealed that it may also be the missing link to chronic inflammation treatment and the start of an exciting new area of treatment for severe, incurable diseases. Nine facts about this powerful bundle of nerves are here.

THE VAGUS NERVE PREVENTS INFLAMMATION

It is common to have a certain level of inflammation following injury or disease. But there are many illnesses and disorders associated with overabundance, ranging from sepsis to acute rheumatoid arthritis. The vagus nerve runs a vast network of fibers around all the organs positioned like spies. When it detects a signal for the initiation of inflammation— the production of cytokines or a substance called the tumor necrosis factor (TNF)—it warns the brain and activates anti-inflammatory neurotransmitters that control the immune response of the body.

Improves Memories

Research by the University of Virginia in rats found that their memory is improved by activating their vagus nerves. Neither the neurotransmitter norepinephrine was released into the amygdale, which preserved memories. Similar trials have been conducted in humans who propose possible therapies for diseases such as Alzheimer's disease.

Increase Respiration

Induced by the vagus nerve, the neurotransmitter acetylcholine signals the lungs to breathe. It is one of the reasons that Botox — often used cosmetically — can be potentially hazardous as it inhibits the production of acetylcholine. Nevertheless, by doing abdominal breathing and holding your breath for four to eight minutes, you can also relax the vagus nerve.

It's Intimately Closely Increase Heart Rate

In the right atrium, where acetylcholine releases slow the pulse, the vagus nerve is responsible for controlling the heart rate through electrical impulses to specialized muscle tissue— the natural pacemaker of the heart. By measuring the time between your heartbeats, and then plotting this on a chart over time, doctors can determine if the heart rate is HRV or variability. This data can provide clues about the resilience of your heart and vagus nerve.

It Increase Body's Sleep/Relaxation Response

The vagus nerve has the brain to calm out by releasing acetylcholine as the ever-vigilant sympathetic nervous system revives the war and flight responses— pouring the stress hormone cortisol and adrenaline into your bloodstream. The tendrils of the vagus nerve penetrate too many muscles, acting like fiber-optic cables that deliver instructions for releasing enzymes and proteins such as prolactin, vasopressin, and oxytocin to calm you down. Upon pain, trauma, or sickness, individuals with a better vagus reaction may be more likely to recover quicker.

It Translates Between the Gut and Brain

The gut makes use of the vagus nerve like a walkie-talkie to communicate with the brain how you feel through "action potentials" electrical impulses.

Overstimulation of the Vagus Nerve Is the Most Common Cause of Fainting

If at the sight of blood you tremble and queasy or get a flu shot, you're not weak. You experience "vagal syncope." Your body stimulates the vagus nerve by responding to stress, causing your blood pressure and heart rate to fall. Blood flow is limited to your brain through intense syncope, and you lose consciousness. But most of the time, for the symptoms to subside, you have to sit down or lie down.

Vagus Nerve Electrical Stimulation Reduces Inflammation Chronic Inflammations and Immune System

Neurosurgeon Kevin Tracey was the first to demonstrate that it could significantly reduce inflammation by activating the vagus nerve. Studies on rats were so good. With stunning results, he repeated the test on humans. For rheumatoid arthritis— which has no known cure and is often treated with toxic drugs — hemorrhagic shock and other equally inflammatory syndromes, the invention of implants to activate the vagus nerve by digital devices shows a drastic reduction and even recovery.

The Vagus Nerve Stimulation Has Created A New Field of Medicine.

An emerging area of medical study, known as bioelectronics, may be the future of medicine, brought on by the popularity of vagal nerve stimulation to combat inflammation and epilepsy. Using electrodes that transmit electrical impulses to different parts of the body, scientists and doctors are trying to treat disease with fewer drugs and fewer side effects.

Digestion microbiome

What is the microbiome?

Most of us humans are bacteria, more than 100 trillion of them. Microbes are more than nine to one of the human cells. Most of them reside in our intestine, particularly in the large intestine. The microbiome is the genetic material of all the microbes-bacteria, fungi, protozoa and viruses-that live on and within the human body.

In the microbiota of one organism, the number of genes in all the bacteria is over 200 times the number of genes in the human genome. The microbiome can weigh up to five pounds.

Microbiome bacteria help digest our food, control our immune system, defend against other disease-causing bacteria, and produce nutrients including B vitamins B12, thiamine and riboflavin, and blood coagulation vitamin K.
There was usually little understanding of the microbiome until the late 1990s.

What does the microbiome have to do with health?

For human development, immunity, and nutrition, the microbiome is essential.
Not invaders, but beneficial colonizers are the bacteria that live in and on us.
Dysfunction in the microbiome is associated with autoimmune diseases such as diabetes, rheumatoid arthritis, muscle dystrophy, multiple sclerosis, and

fibromyalgia. Microbes that cause infection to develop over time, modifying gene expression and metabolic processes, resulting in an unusual immune response to chemicals and tissues that are usually present in the body.

Autoimmune diseases do not seem to be transmitted through inheritance of DNA in families but an inheritance of the microbiome of the body.
Few examples: between overweight and slim twins, the gut microbiome is unique. Obese twins have reduced bacterial diversity and higher enzyme rates, which means that obese twins are more effective in digesting food and calorie production. A bad balance of bacteria in the stomach was also associated with obesity.

Type I diabetes is an autoimmune disease related to a less stable intestinal microbiome. Bacteria play an important role in the development of diabetes in animal studies.

Dust from dog homes can reduce the immune response to allergens and other triggers of asthma by changing the gut microbiome composition. Children living in pet homes are shown to be less likely to develop allergies with kids.

Fecal microbiota transplantation (FMT or fecal transplantation) is a clinical procedure that restores healthy bacteria in the colon by introducing a healthy human donor tool by colonoscopy or enema. Potentially fatal infections with Clostridium Difficile (CDI) are treated using FMT to recover healthy gut microbiota. Colitis, constipation, and irritable bowel syndrome are also treated with FMT.

What is the Human Microbiome Project (HMP)?

The human microbiome is mapped by worldwide scientific projects, giving insight into uncharted species and genomes.
Another project, funded by the National Human Genome Research Institute (NHGRI), part of the

National Institutes of Health (NIH), is the Human Microbiome Project (HMP). The HMP launched as an extension of the Human Genome Project in 2008. It is a five-year feasibility study with a $150 million budget and is being conducted in some centers around the United States.

The HMP aims to research the human being as a supra-organism consisting of non-human and human cells to describe the human microbiome and examine its role in human health and disease.

The HMP's main objective is to classify the metagenome (the aggregate genomes of all microbes) of 300 healthy people's microbiomes across time. A sampling of five areas of the body: hair, mouth, nose, stomach, and vagina.

Why the Human Microbiome important?

The microbiome of a person can affect their susceptibility to infectious diseases and lead to chronic digestive system diseases such as Crohn's disease and irritable bowel syndrome. Many microbe collections decide how a patient responds to drug treatment. The mother's microbiota can affect her children's health.

Scientists studying the human microbiome are finding bacteria and genes that were previously unknown. Genetic studies assessing the relative abundance of different species in the human microbiome have associated specific microbe species combinations with certain aspects of human health.

With a more comprehensive understanding of the diversity of microbes in the human microbiome may lead to new treatments, perhaps by adding more "healthy" bacteria, curing a bacterial infection caused by an "evil" bacterium.

The HMP acts as a guide to define the micro biome's role in wellbeing, diet, immunity, and disease.

What questions remain?

Here are some questions researchers are investigating:

- How is an individual's specific microbiome established? Is this changing over time?
- How does the human host communicate with the microbe community?
- How does a common microbial mix impact nutrition? How are dietary changes impacting the microbiome?
- How does the microbiota affect the immune system and lead to illness?
- How do the bacteria impact the antibiotics? How do the microbes in our bodies affect how we respond to different drugs, on the other hand?
- How to change the microbiota to improve your health?
- And some related ethical issues:
- Is data collected from a valid population sample?
- Sampling approval

- Data sharing and privacy protection
- Sampling invasiveness
- Research results and accidental observations returned to researchers
- Human microbiome test also has broader societal complications:
- How will the research findings be used in clinical settings?
- How to control new products such as probiotics?
- How will the public perceive microbiome discoveries?
- How could this knowledge alter health and disease definitions, including what it means to be human?

Nerve stimulation may improve sexuality

The electrodes are not the first thing most people think about when it comes to sexual excitement. But if any signs may quickly change the results of a pilot study.

Female sexual dysfunction (FSD), a disorder ranging from lack of libido to orgasm failure, affects 40% to 45% of women, particularly as they age.

FSD can be difficult to diagnose and even harder to treat.

And while doctors have tried to help women by administering sildenafil (better known by its brand name, Viagra), these approaches do not always work with hormones, so flibanserin and may have unwanted side effects.

VAGUS NERVE AND ANXIETY

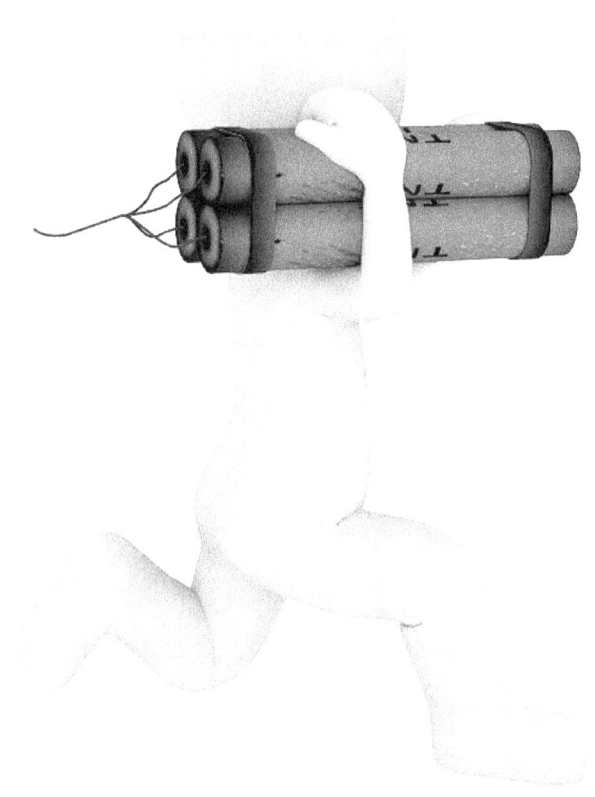

The vagus nerve is the tenth of 12 cranial nerve pairs and the longest in the body. Also, in Latin, the word vagus means "vagabond," and perfectly illustrates the direction of this nerve which spreads through different body organs.

In the cranial bag, precisely in the spinal cord, the vagus nerve is born and slides into the neck which grows on two branches and enters the stomach which travels along the way through the different organs.

The vagus nerve interferes with the development of the mucous membranes of the respiratory system and transmits the breathing rhythm, power and speed. It affects the pharynx, larynx, esophagus, trachea, and bronchi, as well as cardiac, stomach, pancreatic, and liver nerve fibers. But it also conducts the opposite mission; that is, it collects signals from the internal organs and sends them for transmission to the brain.

But perhaps the most interesting thing is the relationship between the vagus nerve and fear, as it also transmits tense and relaxed, rage and calming signals.

To understand the connection between the vagus nerve and fear, we need to recognize that there are two "opposite" mechanisms in the nervous system that continuously send information to the brain.

They are primed for action by the sympathetic nervous system, so it primarily supplies hormones including adrenaline and cortisol. During rest and relaxation, the parasympathetic nervous system interferes.

These systems work as accelerators and decelerators in operation. The sympathetic nervous system speeds up and stimulates us as the parasympathetic nervous system makes us calm and decrease volume, so it uses neurotransmitters such as acetylcholine, and reduces heart rate and blood pressure and allow the muscles function faster.

The functions of the vagus nerve

The parasympathetic system is controlled by the vagus nerve. This interferes with many processes, from mouth to breathing, and it can also cause various effects when it is affected. Some of the body's vagus nerve functions are:

- It helps regulate rhythm, regulates muscle movements, and keeps breathing rate.
- Maintains the operation of the digestive tract, facilitating the absorption of food by the contraction of the stomach and intestine muscles.
- It facilitates relief after a stressful situation and reveals that we are in danger and need not lower the guard.
- Return sensory information about the state of the body to the cortex.

Vagus nerve and anxiety

The sympathetic nervous system is triggered when we are exposed to stressful situations. If the stress continues and we are unable to shut off the physiological response that causes it, it will not be long before problems appear. This includes triggering two pathways at the brain level: the hypothalamus-pituitary-adrenal axis and the axis of the brain-intestine.

The brain responds to stress and anxiety by enhancing the production of hormones (CRFs) that migrate from the hypothalamus to the pituitary gland where they trigger the release of another hormone (ACTH), which in effect travels through the bloodstream to the adrenal glands to promote the activation of cortisol and adrenaline, which serve as suppressors of the immune system and inflammatory precursors.

And as if that were not enough, there is a rise in glutamate in the brain caused by chronic stress and anxiety, a neurotransmitter that triggers migraine, depression and anxiety when produced in abundance. Additionally, a high cortisol level decreases the hippocampus size, the part of the brain that is responsible for creating new memories.

Vagus nerve activity can result in signs such as dizziness, gastrointestinal problems, arrhythmias, respiratory difficulties, and excessive emotional responses. Besides, since the vagus nerve cannot activate the relaxing signal, the sympathetic nervous system remains active, this will cause the patient to respond impulsively and suffer from anxiety.

It is also interesting that a study at Miami University showed that the vagal tone is being passed from mother to child. People with fear, stress or a lot of anger during gestation had a lower vagal activity and their babies also had higher vagal activity and lower dopamine and serotonin rates.

3 vagal stimulation techniques: how to take care of the vagus nerve?

The vagal tone is an intrinsic biological process reflecting the vagus nerve function. The rise in vagal tone stimulates the parasympathetic nervous system, indicating that after a stressful situation, we will recover quicker and this will have a positive impact on our emotional balance and overall health.

There are different techniques for relaxing the vagus nerves:

Exposure to cold

Exposure to cold has been seen to activate the vagus nerve as it activates the cholinergic neurons that cross these innervations. Nevertheless, an investigation at the University of Oulu has shown that regular cold exposure helps to reduce the reaction to fight-flight, which activates the sympathetic nervous system.

A cold shower for 30 seconds per day or a warm towel on the head can be enough. Some lay on the belly and place a block of ice on the nape. Some want a glass of cold water to drink easily.

Diaphragmatic breathing

Many people inhale 10 to 14 times a minute of air, which ensures they have a shallow pulse. The goal would be six times a minute to inhale water. Another very effective method for vagal relaxation is, therefore, to breathe deeply.

In particular, diaphragmatic breathing activates the vagus nerve, and the brain interprets it as having to calm down, even though the nerve has not specifically given that order. The process is the same for which you will experience brief flashes of light as you close your eyes and click your fingertips on your eyelids because they are perceived by the brain.

They allow a deeper breath with diaphragmatic breathing which takes oxygen into the lower part of the lungs, properly using the diaphragm and encouraging relaxing.

Meditation, yoga and tai-chi

Meditation can improve the tone of the vagus. This has been shown by Oregon University researchers who have seen that only five days of meditation in mindfulness encourage positive feelings about themselves which induce vagus nerve stimulation, thus modulating the function of the parasympathetic nervous system, a much better result than traditional methods for calming.

DEPRESSION (MAJOR DEPRESSIVE DISORDER)

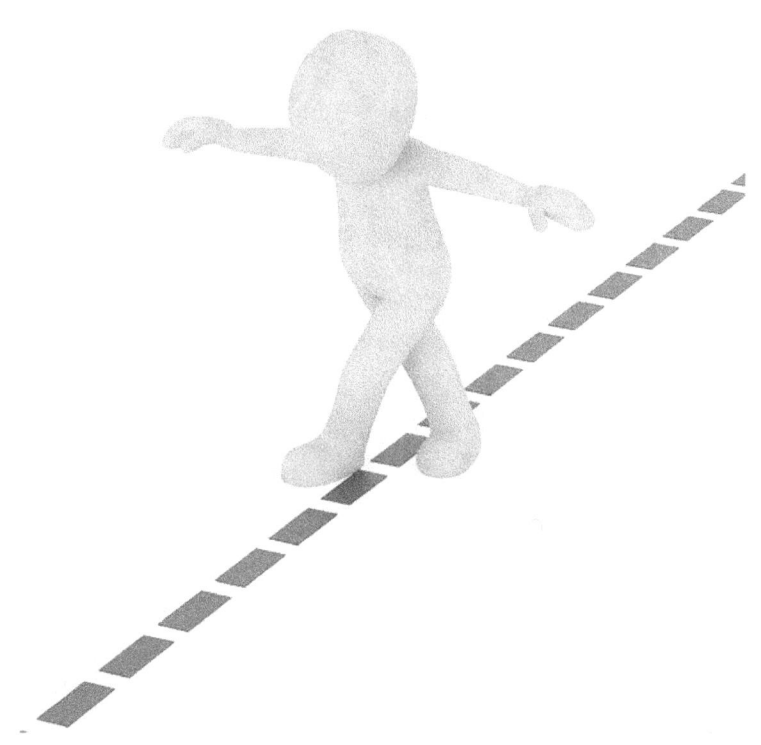

Depression is a mood disorder that causes continuous sadness or loss of interest. Often known as major depressive disorder or clinical depression, it affects how you look, think and act, and can contribute to a variety of physical or emotional problems. You may have difficulty completing normal daily activities, and you may often feel like life isn't worth living.

Depression is not a flaw, more than just a case of blues, and you can't just "snap out" of it. Depression can require treatment in the long term. But don't be disheartened. Through medicine, psychotherapy or both, most people with depression feel better.

Symptoms

Because during your lifespan depression can happen only once, people usually experience multiple episodes. Symptoms occur most of the day, nearly every day, during these events, and may include:

- Feelings of sadness or hopelessness
- Irritability or frustration
- Loss of interest
- Insomnia
- Tiredness

- Appetite and weight loss
- Anxiety
- Restlessness
- Slowed thinking
- Feelings of worthlessness
- Self-blame
- Overthinking
- Suicidal thoughts

Symptoms are usually severe enough for many people with depression to cause significant problems in day-to-day activities such as work, school, social activities, or relationships with others. Most people may feel sad or depressed in particular without really knowing why.

Depression symptoms in children and teens

Some signs and symptoms of depression are close to those of adults in children and adolescents, but some variations can occur.

- Symptoms of depression in younger children may include fatigue, irritability, cramping,

- panic, nausea, reluctance to go to school, or underweight.
- In teens, symptoms may include depression, irritability, feeling pessimistic or meaningless, frustration, poor performance or poor attendance at school, feeling confused or extremely sensitive, eating and sleeping too much, losing interest in normal activities, and avoiding social contact.

Depression symptoms in older adults

Depression is not a natural part of growing older, nor should it be taken lightly. Unfortunately, anxiety in older adults sometimes remains undiagnosed and untreated and may be hesitant to seek assistance. Symptoms of depression in older adults can be different or less apparent, such as:

- Memory disturbances and changes in personality
- Physical impairment and discomfort

- Tiredness, lack of appetite, sleep problems and loss of interest in sex— not induced by a medical condition or treatment
- Always wanting to stay at home, rather than socializing or doing new things
- Suicidal thoughts and emotions, especially in older people.

When to see a doctor

When you feel depressed, make an appointment as soon as possible to see a doctor or mental health specialist. If you are unwilling to seek help, speak to a friend or loved one, any health care provider, a person of faith, or someone else you know.

Should you think you might injure yourself and try to commit suicide, call your local emergency line.

If you have suicidal thoughts, consider those choices as well:

- Call your doctor or professionals in the field of mental health.
- Dial a hotline number for a suicide

- Contact a trusted friend or loved one.
- Consult a spiritual leader or someone else in your faith community.

If you have a loved one who is in danger of suicide or has made a suicide attempt, make sure someone remains with that person — call your local emergency line immediately. But, if you think you can do so safely, take the person to the closest hospital emergency room.

Causes

Just what causes anxiety is not understood. Like many mental disorders, it may include a variety of factors, such as:

- **Biological differences.** People with depression in their bodies seem to have physical changes. The meaning of these changes is still uncertain, but it may ultimately help to identify causes.
- **Chemistry of the brain.** Neurotransmitters are brain chemicals that occur naturally and

are likely to play a role in depression. Recent research shows that improvements in the action and effect of these neurotransmitters and how they interact with neurocircuits involved in maintaining mood control may play a major role in depression and recovery.
- **Hormones.** Changes in the hormone balance of the body can cause or trigger depression. Increases in hormones can arise from pregnancy and thyroid problems, menopause or a variety of other conditions during the weeks or months of childbirth (postpartum).
- **Traits inherited.** Depression is more common in people who also have this condition in their blood relatives. Scientists are trying to find mutations that can cause depression.

Risk factors

Depression mostly begins in teenagers, twenties or thirties, but it can occur at any age. Depression is associated with more women than men, but this may be partly due to women being more likely to seek care.

Factors that tend to increase the risk that depression can grow or cause include:

- Certain personality traits, such as low self-esteem and being too dependent, self-critical or pessimistic
- Traumatic or stressful events, such as physical or sexual abuse, death or loss of a loved one, difficult relationships or financial problems
- Blood relatives with a history of depression, bipolar disorder, alcoholism or suicide
- Being homosexual, gay, bisexual and transgender and possessing differences in the production of genital organs that are not distinctly male or female (intersex) in an unsupportive environment
- Experience of other mental health disorders such as anxiety disorder, eating disorders and post-traumatic stress disorder.

- Alcohol addiction and illicit drugs
- Chronic illnesses, including diabetes, stroke, chronic pain and heart disease
- Other medications, such as high blood pressure medicines and sleeping pills (talk to your doctor before quitting medicines)

Complications

Depression is a serious disorder that can pay you and your family a terrible price. Depression often gets worse if it is not treated, leading to emotional, behavioral and health issues affecting every area of your life.

Examples of depression-related complications include:

- Overweight that can lead to heart disease or diabetes
- Pain and physical illness
- Drug and drug abuse
- Depression, panic disorder and social phobia

- Family issues, marriage challenges and struggles with work or school
- Social alienation
- Suicidal thoughts, suicide attempts and suicide
- Self-mutilation as a result of medical conditions
- Premature death

Prevention

- Take steps to manage stress, improve tolerance and increase self-esteem.
- Involve family and friends, especially in times of turmoil, to help you survive raw spells.
- Seek medication at the first indication of a problem to help prevent the escalation of depression.
- Seek therapy and long-term care to help prevent symptoms from returning.

VAGUS NERVE IN MEDITATION

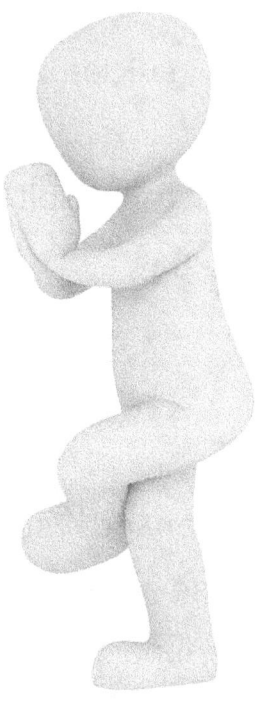

The Vagus Nerve is associated with mindfulness. The roughly translated vagus nerve means "walking cord." This travels from the brain stem to the stomach and interacts with many of the major organs involved in many of our body functions such as breathing, feeding, heart rate, and much more.

It is intimately connected to the autonomic (automatic) nervous system's parasympathetic branch and thus plays a major role in controlling stress. The autonomic nervous system naturally controls our bodies without our intervention. Functions such as heart rate are an artificial nervous system feature.

There are two branches of the autonomic nervous system, the sympathetic and the parasympathetic. The supportive branch is responsible for bringing us into combat or flight, and the parasympathetic branch is responsible for taking us out of battle or flight and controlling our bodies if not engaged in a fight or flight situation.

Stress levels are at historic highs, and the patterns of getting stuck in fight or flight are one of the reasons for this. Our nervous systems are trapped in the protective state for many reasons, meaning that the changes that take place in our body/mind during battle and flight will not be reversed after the event occurs. Such improvements also stick with us for extended periods in varying degrees. This results in chronic stress leading to a host of signs of physical, emotional, and emotion.

Research has provided us with many tools to test different body functions and assess levels of stress. Studying the activation of the Vagus Nerve is one of the most powerful ways of measuring these stress levels. When activated by the Vagus Nerve, it stimulates the autonomic nervous system's parasympathetic branch to come out of fight or flight, thus reducing stress. Via mindfulness, this is how it happens.

We know that meditation is successful in lowering stress, particularly meditation on consciousness (full attention to the present moment). Mindfulness meditation is the most studied approach to mindfulness, having conducted more than 2,500 articles worldwide, with an average of an estimated 200 per month. I find it to be the core of the mindfulness cycle, strengthening all the other approaches to meditation and being a stand-alone exercise itself. Such findings show that meditation can increase energy, decrease pressure, slow breathing, decrease depression, decrease pain, increase blood flow and provide a sense of peace to name a few. When the Vagus Nerve absorbs the messages from these effects of relaxation, it sends a message to the brain that everything is well, there is no risk, and there is no need for battle or flight. The brain then sends the message to the autonomous nervous system which activates the parasympathetic component to emerge from battle and flight and to maintain the processes in equilibrium. This is an example of functioning together between the Vagus Nerve and the heart. The mind will send messages through the Vagus Nerve to the body and the body to the heart.

It is interesting to note that, in reality, a feature of the body previously thought to operate automatically can be deliberately affected by meditation. This is very important and gives us insight into the possibility of participating in our health and well-being consciously in many ways.

This is yet another example of the relation between mind and body and how our feelings, impulses and physical sensations are intertwined and how mindfulness can make the system run smoothly.

Reducing Stress with Sensate

Forget meditation. Forget about yoga every day. There's a clever new pressure-busting device soon hitting the market that can be the best way to reduce long-term stress and anxiety, and working on your vagus nerve is all about. Starting with the brain stem, the vagus nerve passes through the throat to the heart, lungs and diaphragm, before spreading root-like diversity into the intestine.

The vagus nerve is quite important as it controls our reaction to our senses, which makes it remarkable that so little attention has been paid to it—so far. It manages the battle and flight process as our stress superhighway, and in this age of constant communication and fast-paced life, current stress levels mean the vagus is overworked for many.

Evidence demonstrates that using low-frequency soundwaves to actively activate the vagus nerve puts the brakes on the reaction to stress, which in effect helps to regulate stress levels. Vagus nerve stimulation therapies successfully reduce heart rate, decrease blood pressure and breathing rates, and aid metabolism, reducing stress levels to heal the body.

Throughout Scandinavia, vagal toning has been commonly used where it is referred to as vibroacoustic therapy and where it is known that it has helped speed up recovery rates from chronic anxiety and stress-related diseases. Migraine also aids. The U.S. military used vagal toning on Iraq-backed troops suffering from PTSD and recorded a 97 percent reduction in levels of depression.

Move into the Sensate. A pebble-shaped device equipped for low-frequency sound waves to activate the vagus nerve which can be changed in strength using your smartphone. It must be positioned on the breastbone where the nerve is closer to the ground and can be worn next to the skin or over the dress. Trials prove this helps to reduce stress levels effectively, and the use of just ten minutes per day can create a phenomenal improvement in overwhelming stress levels.

The Sensate will have different programs based on whether you need simple stress relief, focus support, or sleep assistance. This is going to be a real winner for those who consider mindfulness applications that are less than calming. It's not cheap, usually priced at £199.99, but due to stress, it causes premature ageing along with a host of other medical issues that most believe will sign up immediately.

The Sensate may be the fast path to a stress-free state, but there are other techniques for vagus toning to try:

Belly Breathing

Push your tummy out as you breathe in through your nose (there is a tendency to hold it in). Count for five, then rapidly exhale through the nose. The vagus nerve starts with a slow, abdominal deep breathing kick and helps to relieve stress and insomnia.

Singing

The vocal cords vibrate, which in turn stimulates the vagus. Not because of you? Then it may be more compelling to sing. A deep guttural vibrates on the back of the throat where the nerve of the vagus ends. Likewise, gargling will have the same result for just one minute.

PHYSIOLOGICAL BENEFITS OF MEDITATION

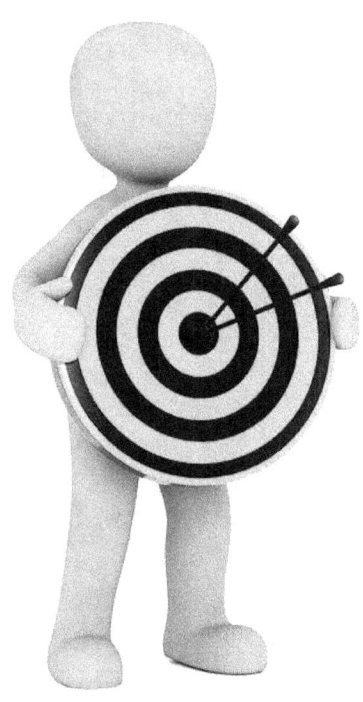

It is no surprise that in Western traditions, mindfulness has its main origins. In reality, it can date meditation as far back as 5000 B.C. In the Hindu revolution. But in many religious traditions, including Christianity and Islam, the practice of meditation can be found. We know it as "prayer" in Christianity, especially the ritualistic prayer forms such as the rosary and Catholic adoration. As late as 1975, John Main, Benedictine monk, re-introduced a method of meditation marked by a prayer-phrase repeated chant. The World Christian Meditation Group was founded in 1991.

New Age, the outgrowth of hippie-counterculture and the astrological emergence of the' 60s and' 70s' Age of Aquarius, synthesized contemporary Western theories of medicine (psychology) and evolution with Yoga, Hinduism, and Buddhism. Since New Age is more of an individualized religious movement than organized religion, it contributed significantly to a wider, more modern tolerance and mindfulness practice. Increasing awareness and affirmation of the benefits of Yoga has resulted in a growing number of secularized training centres for Yoga, not so much as a religious practice as a body/mind fitness regime. Apart from their physical exercise courses, most health and wellness clubs offer yoga fitness classes. My wife is a Body Training Systems (BTS) accredited trainer named Team Centergy, a Thai-chi Yoga and Pilates synthesis. As a product of pure correlation, the increased popularity of yoga and its symbiotic relationship with meditation has led to the increased secularization and identification with meditation in the context of contemporary western society.

With the ever-increasing awareness of lifestyle, psychological stress and its negative side effects on health and longevity, scientific sciences have taken a closer look at meditation's long-professed benefits. This was followed by increased interest in and adoption of traditional non-western medicine (sometimes included in the "alternative medicine" category). Scientific comparisons between the reduction of muscle tension and reduction of depression were created by the Western physicians of the 1920s. A medical treatise on Spiritual relaxation techniques to reduce stress and chronic pain, Dr. Ainslie Meares wrote Recovery Without

Drugs in the 1960s. Dr. Herbert Benson published The Relaxation Response in 1975, an extension of the same subject. Today, in Western psychology and psychotherapy philosophies, yoga meditation is popular. But more importantly, more and more scientific evidence of the therapeutic benefits of meditation is being sought in medical research.

We understand that unnecessary physical and psychological stress can have negative effects on our health and longevity in the short and long term. Our contemporary culture is constantly finding ways to "decompress." But it's hard to find the "downtime" from the negative stressors of our modern lifestyles under increased two-income family financial stresses. Of note, short-term relaxation is offered by weekend breaks from our multi-tasking lives. And the yearly holiday to the tropics ' slower pace (if we can afford it) can take a while to reduce our blood pressure. But how often do we learn of a friend who came back more tired from their holidays than when they left. It seems that we are so used in our activity-packed lives that even when we leave, we continue to schedule our vacations as if we were in one of those shopping spree competitions, racing frenziedly from one tourist attraction to another to ensure that we get the most of our time.

The question is, how can we in our daily lives reduce and counteract the effects of stress?

There are regular constructive de-stressing techniques. For example, the effects of dancing, smiling, and mindfulness are supported by scientific medical evidence. Not only can these behaviors reduce stress, they can also improve the immune system dramatically. For simplicity's sake, let's find the meditation's physiological effects.

In accordance with our vagus nerve, the main controller for disease in our major organs, our brain responds to pressure as if the pathogen cells of a bacterial attack are identified. If you had an infected wound on your thumb, the response of mind and body is to send white blood cells to combat the infection war. Our finger is turning red, swelling, and radiating heat at the point of the cut inflames. The vagus nerve can over-react to pressure, prompting the brain to protect our primary organs and cardiovascular system.

Once our vagus nerve senses stress-related discomfort in muscles, it signals the brain to send troops to fight the war as if we had an attacking virus, just as our immune system would demand a response to our finger's contaminated wound. This leads not only to increased stomach acid and inflammation, but also to inflammation of our artery linings, which makes us more susceptible to arterial sclerosis and stroke.

Meditation has been found to help relax the overly reactive vagus nerve and shut down the physiological response caused by stress by these forms of inflammation. The pressure is not removed by mindfulness. It soothes our physiological stress reaction. It can also lower our pain levels.

We know for sure that our body needs good quality oxygen-rich air to work at its best. Football fans saw players sitting on the sidelines breathing additional oxygen to recover their exhausted oxygen due to physical exertion demands, especially in higher-altitude cities like Denver. You may have noted that through their nose the players inhale deeply. Long-distance runners inhale through their nose and exhale through their mouth to increase stamina and endurance. Clearly, with our nose, we should be able to inhale much more water (and oxygen). So why inhaling through their nose will help a distance runner or a tired football player? This is not because of an increase in oxygen intake, but because of an increase in nitric oxide (NO), which helps blood vessels to expand and dilate, thereby improving the total blood flow. We know little about this very critical yet ephemeral gas (it is just seconds in lifespan), which plays a major role in our body functions. Nitric oxide is absorbed only by the lining of our nasal passages, usually in small percentages of the air we breathe. Because our body has a very short lifespan, we need to replenish it by breathing through our nose as often and as profoundly as we can.

Many breathing techniques promote intense nose inhalation and mouth exhalation. This seems to have very positive effects on the regeneration and rejuvenation of organ function, particularly in relation to the cardiovascular system. Enhanced nitric oxide absorption by meditative deep breathing functions as a neurotransmitter in the brain, similar to serotonin and dopamine, providing a calming effect in reducing stress and encouraging awakening. Therefore, immediately after waking from sleep, this form of meditation is best practiced. In contrast, nitric oxide promotes healthy skin and decreases hair loss.

Meditation may not be a remedy for baldness, but there is substantial evidence that its advantages of stress reduction and increased blood flow greatly lead to increased resistance to disease and reducing heart inflammation. Heart surgeons recommend therapy more frequently to their patients as part of the post-surgery protocol.

VAGUS NERVE EXERCISES

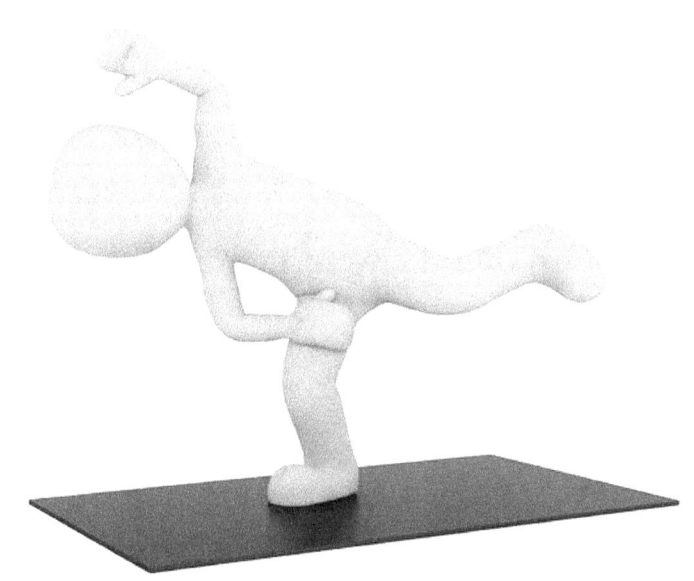

- Turn on neurogenesis, allowing our brains to sprout new cells of the brain.
- Through the relaxing response, shut off stress, hyper-arousal, and fight/flight.
- Our memories sharpen.
- Combat the infection or inflammation.

- Allow you to tolerate high blood pressure.
- Block cortisol hormone and other oxidizing agents that degrade and deteriorate the brain and body.
- Block systemic (body-wide) inflammation–a major factor in aging and poor health.
- Help us to conquer anxiety and depression.
- Help us get to rest.
- Raise human growth hormone levels.
- Help them overcome resistance to insulin.
- Discard allergic reactions.
- Lower chances of stress and headaches of tension.
- Help save and expand our mitochondria— this is key to keeping our energy levels optimum and not damaging our DNA and RNA.
- It influences our general ability to live shorter, happier and more active lives.

How to Activate the Vagus Nerve on Your Own?

A variety of meditation and calming strategies can easily turn on vagus nerve stimulation:

- 'OM ' Chanting
- Coldwater face immersion during exercise
- Fill the mouth with saliva and submerge the tongue to induce a hyper-relaxing vagal reaction.
- Inhale through your nose and exhale through your mouth to practice deep breathing.
- Breathe faster.
- Breathe harder from the belly.
- Breathe out faster than you breathe in.

You can learn how to use breathing exercises to shift your focus away from pain. One thing at a time is handled by the human mind. When you concentrate on your breathing pattern, the pain is not the priority. Most of us tend to stop breathing and hold our breath as we anticipate pain.

Breath-holding stimulates the reaction to fight/flight/freeze; it tends to increase discomfort, weakness, panic, and terror perception.

You can proceed as follows: take a deep inhalation (i.e., expanding your diaphragm) into your belly to the count of five, pause, and then slowly exhale through a small hole in your mouth. Most people take about 10 to 14 breaths per minute while they are at rest. To enter parasympathetic/relaxation/healing mode, lowering the pulse to 5-7 times per minute is best. Exhaling through your eyes instead of the nose makes your breathing more aware and lets you to effectively detect your breath. When you lower your breaths every minute and enter the parasympathetic mode, your muscles will relax and decrease your anxieties and worries. The delivery of oxygen to the cells of your body increases, helping to produce endorphins, the feel-good molecules of the brain. For decades, Tibetan monks have been doing' conscious meditation,' but it is not a secret. By imagining that you inhale IN love, you can enhance your experience and exhale

OUT gratitude. Such ancient strategies will also strengthen your brain, battle anxiety, lower blood pressure, and heart rate and raise your immune systems — and it's safe!

'OM' Chanting

In 2011, the International Journal of Yoga published an interesting study in which' OM' chanting was correlated with' SSS' pronunciation as well as a rest state to decide if chanting is more appealing to the vagus nerve. The study found the chanting to be more effective than either the pronunciation of' sss' or the state of rest. Effective ' OM' chanting is linked to a sensation of vibration around the ears and throughout the body. Such a sensation is also expected to be transmitted through the auricular branch of the vagus nerve and will result in the deactivation of the limbic (HPA axis).

How can I chant?

Hold the' OM' part of the vowel (o) for 5 seconds and proceed for the next 10 seconds into the consonant (m) part. Proceed to chant for ten minutes. Start with a deep breath and start in appreciation.

Cold Water

Physical exercise leads to increased sympathetic activation (HPA axis— combat/flight, pressure response), along with parasympathetic withdrawal (rest, sleep, regeneration, immune system), resulting in a higher heart rate (HR). Studies have found that cold water face immersion tends to be a simple and efficient way of promoting parasympathetic reactivation directly following exercise through the vagus nerve, enhancing heart rate reduction, intestinal motility, and turning on the immune system on. In a non-exercise setting, triggering the vagus nerve is also active.

Subjects remained seated in hot-water face immersion and bent their heads forward into a cold-water tub. The mask is soaked to submerge the nose, mouth, and at least two-thirds of the two cheeks.

The temperature of the air was set at 10 12 ° C.

Increased Salivation

The more relaxed the mind and the greater the tension, the faster the salivation stimulus will be. You know that the Vagus Nerve has been activated, and the body is in parasympathetic mode when the mouth can produce large quantities of saliva.

Try to relax and recline in a chair to stimulate salivation and imagine a juicy lemon. Just rest your tongue in this bath as your mouth fills with saliva (if this doesn't happen, fill your mouth with a small amount of warm water and rest your tongue in this bath. Just relaxing will stimulate saliva secretion). Relax and enjoy your arms, feet, knees, neck, back and head relaxed. Breathe this feeling profoundly and remain here as long as you can.

METHOD TO ACTIVATE VAGUS NERVE

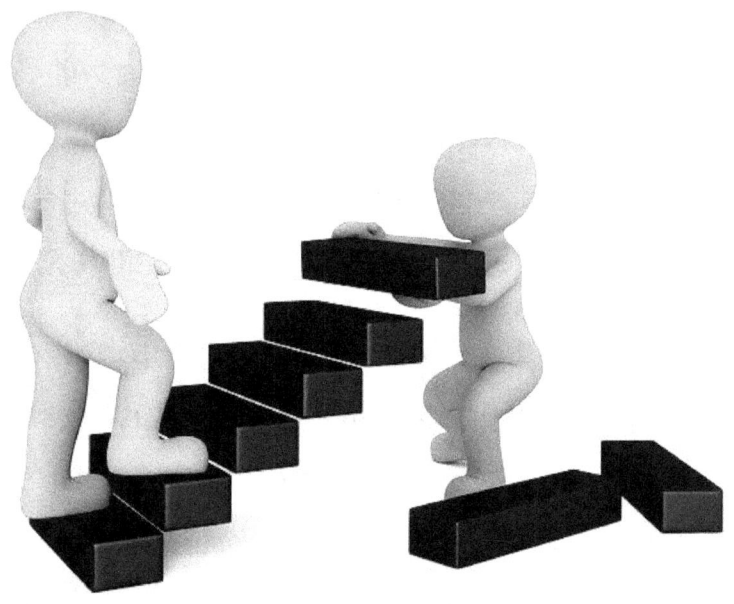

The 10th of the cranial nerves, it is often called the "Nerve of Compassion" because when it is active, it helps to create the "warm-fuzziness" that we feel in our chest when we get a hug or are moved by something... The vagus nerve is a bundle of nerves that originates at the top of the spinal cord. It activates various organs (such as the heart, lungs, liver, and digestive organs) throughout the body. If alive, the sensation of hot expansion in the chest is likely to be produced — for example, when we are moved by the goodness of somebody or when we enjoy a lovely piece of music.

Long ago, neuroscientist Stephen W. Porges of Chicago's University of Illinois argued that the vagus nerve is[the compassion nerve] (of course, it also serves many other functions). This argument was supported by several reasons. It is believed that the vagus nerve in the vocal chamber activates other muscles, facilitating contact. It decreases the heart rate. Some new science shows that oxytocin, a neurotransmitter implicated in trust and maternal attachment, may be closely linked to receptor networks.

Our research and that of other scientists suggest that vagus nerve activation is associated with care feelings and the ethical intuition that common humanity is shared by people from different social groups (even adversarial ones). We also found that people with high vagus nerve activation are prone to feelings, feelings that foster altruism—compassion, empathy, affection, and joy.

Psychologist Nancy Eisenberg has shown that it is more supportive and likely to give children with high-baseline vagus nerve involvement. This area of study is the beginning of a fascinating new altruism argument: that a part of our nervous system has developed to promote such behavior.

STRESS & THE VAGUS NERVE

The autonomic nervous system (ANS) regulates the levels of stress hormones in your body. The ANS has two components, the sympathetic nervous system (SNS) and the parasympathetic nervous system (PNS), which balance one another.

Your nervous system turns up the SNS. It helps us manage what we perceive to be emergencies and is responsible for the response of flight.

The PNS turns the nervous system down and helps us to calm down. This encourages relaxation, rest, sleep, and drowsiness by slowing down our heart rate, slowing down our breathing, limiting our eyes' pupils, increasing our mouth's saliva production, and so on.

The vagus nerve is the brain-derived nerve that controls the parasympathetic nervous system that controls your response to relaxation. The neurotransmitter is used by this nervous system, acetylcholine. If your brain is unable to interact with your diaphragm by the vagus nerve release of acetylcholine (e.g., affected by botulinum toxin), then you will stop breathing and die.

Training and learning are important for acetylcholine. It is also soothing and stimulating the vagus nerve uses to transmit healing and relaxation signals across the body. New research has found a significant brake on inflammation in the body by acetylcholine. Stimulating the vagus nerve, in other words, releases acetylcholine across the skin, not only calming but also turning down the inflammatory flames that are associated with the harmful effects of stress.

Exciting new work has also connected the vagus nerve to enhanced neurogenesis, increased BDNF production (neurotrophic brain-derived factor is like super fertilizer for your brain cells) and brain tissue recovery, and real body-wide regeneration.

HEALTH, LONGEVITY & AGING

As you get older, more inflammatory molecules are released by your immune system, and your nervous system flips on the stress response, causing deterioration and aging of the body.

It's not just talking. Scientific studies support it.

For instance, Feinstein Institute for Medical Research's director, Kevin Tracey, discovered how the brain controls the immune system through a direct nerve-based connection.

He defines this as the reaction of inflammation I put, and this is the response of the immune system to the brain.

Let me describe it to you.

A muscle called the vagus nerve regulates the immune system.

But it's not just a nerve.

It is the brain's most powerful nerve, and it connects to all the major organs.

And you can stimulate this nerve— through mindfulness, meditation, and other ancient exercises, such as the Light Language Mayan system, together with the Team & Steve Rother's new vagus nerve stimulation methods, the vagus nerve can be triggered and activated by rhythm, amplitude, color, and light.

What's the benefit of that?
You can regulate the immune cells by stimulating the vagus nerve, reducing inflammation, and even preventing disease and aging!

That's true. You can turn on the vagus nerve to control anxiety by creating positive brain cycles—as the yoga masters have done for centuries.

Through this method, you can control your gene function. Activate the vagus nerve and the genes that help control the inflammation can be switched on. Inflammation is one of disease and aging's key factors.

CELLULAR REGENERATION

The discovery that our bodies can regenerate at any age has been even more fascinating.

Yale University's Diane Krause, MD, Ph.D., discovered that our innate adult stem cells (cells that can turn from our bone marrow into any cell in the body) could be transformed into liver, intestine, lung, and skin cells. It's a fantastic breakthrough. This is why.

This means we will create new cells and at any point, regenerate our organs and tissues.

And how are they regulated by these stem cells?

You guessed: the nerve of the vagus.

For example, stem cells are shown to be directly connected to the vagus nerve by Theise et al. Activating the vagus nerve will activate stem cells to produce or restore new cells or regenerate your organs.

So relaxation— a state of calm, harmony, and quietness— can stimulate the nerve of the vagus.

And also, the vagus nerve stimulates your stem cells to rebuild your tissues and organs and renew them.

Scientists have even demonstrated how meditation increases and improves the brain. Through getting into the laboratory Tibetan lamas skilled in attention and mind regulation, they worked out the brain function of "qualified mediators."

Among mediators, they found higher concentrations of gamma brain waves and thinner cortexes of the brain (the regions associated with higher brain function).

Other strong effects that relaxation can have on our physiology.

In ecology, safety needs to be a complex system that can respond to its environment and is robust and versatile.

The same happens to us.

The happier we are, the most dynamic and robust we are.

Take our heartbeat, for instance.

Its complexity is called variability in heart rate (HRV) or variability in beat-to-beat. The happier you are, the more complex the HRV is. The worst heart rate is the least dynamic — a flat line.

So what does relaxation have to do with this?

The vagus nerve also controls the HRV.

As you can see, turning on the response to relaxation and activating the vagus nerve is essential for health.

Activating the Vagus Nerve Will:
- Reduce inflammation
- Help your organs and cells to regenerate by activating stem cells
- Increase heart rate variability
- Thicken your brain (which normally decreases with aging).
- Modify your nervous system
- Reduce depression and stress
- Improve performance
- Improve the quality of life

COMPASSION & DNA

Elizabeth Blackburn, Ph.D., who invented telomeres, explained that they gradually become so small that our DNA ends up unraveling and that we can no longer reproduce our cells, and we die.

Remarkably, mental stress allows the telomeres to shorten more rapidly — which results in accelerated aging.

What's more amazing than that?

The health of the caregivers' telomeres was determined by their behavior in a sample of caregivers with sick patients!

It does not sound possible, but it is real.

The nurses who thought the treatment was a strain had shorter telomeres, while there was no shortening for those who viewed their work as a chance to be caring.

The Dalai Lama said the compassion seat is, in fact, biological and — necessary to survive.

Perhaps the real secret for survival is the creation of empathy and experience in dealing with difficult living conditions.

It may just be that engaging with constructive methods such as yoga and similar techniques to recognize our true nature is vital for health and longevity by nurturing our minds and hearts.

By changing our minds, the ways we can change our bodies is no longer a theory.

A new scientific vocabulary is available to explain how the mind's characteristics influence the body through effects on the vagus nerve, immune cells, stem cells, telomeres, Rna, and more.

Note, to self-regulate, heal, rebuild, and survive, and the body has all the tools and endlessly adaptable mechanisms.

You need to learn how to work with your body, not against it. Then you can have a happy, prosperous life–and spend your entire lifetime, which can be as high as 120 + years!

SOUND THERAPY AS MEDICINE TO STIMULATE THE VAGUS NERVE

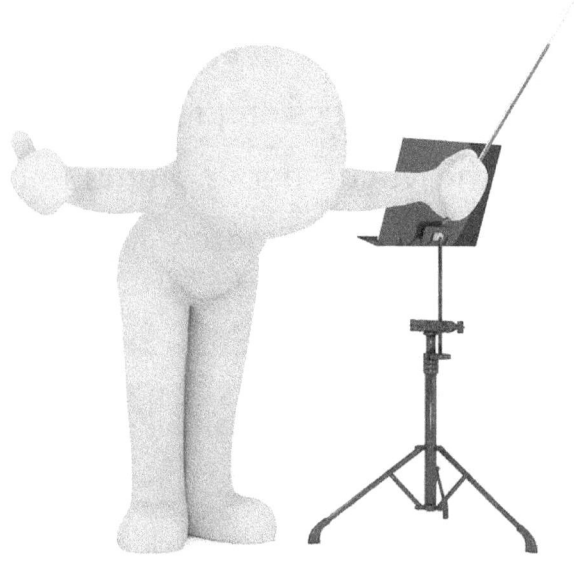

The vagus nerve is important when it comes to mind-body contact, as it enters all the major organs except the adrenal and thyroid glands.

This is an essential nerve for any organ with which it is in contact. It's what allows the mind to suppress anxiety and depression. Whether they communicate with each other is closely related to the nerve of the vagus as it is connected to the nerves that guide our ears for speech, it controls eye contact and those that control gestures. This nerve also can influence the proper release of hormones in the body which keeps our mental and physical processes balanced.

For ease of digestion in the stomach, it is the vagus nerve responsible for increasing stomach acidity and digestive juice secretion. It may also allow you to digest vitamin B12 when activated. If it doesn't work properly, then you can expect serious intestinal problems like colitis, IBS, or Re-flux, to name a few. Re-flux problems are caused by a vagus nerve problem because the oesophagus is also regulated by it. It is the oesophagus' unsuitable reflex that triggers disorders such as Gerd and Re-flux.

The vagus nerve also helps to control blood pressure and heart rate, stopping heart disease. While it is this nerve that regulates the balance of blood glucose in the liver and pancreas, avoiding diabetes, the vagus nerve helps release bile when it passes through the gallbladder, which is what helps your body eliminate toxins and break down fat. While in the bladder, this nerve facilitates the general activity of the kidney, increasing blood flow, enhancing filtration of our bodies. When the vagus nerve enters the spleen, activation in all target organs may reduce inflammation. Even this nerve has the power to control women's fertility and orgasms. A vagus nerve that is disabled or blocked can cause havoc throughout the mind and body.

Now that we realize that the vagus nerve is connected to all the major organs and their proper functioning, we can easily conclude that by triggering and relaxing the vagus nerve, any illness, infection or disease of the brain, heart, and spirit can be reversed or even healed. So you will also have positive effects on issues such as anxiety disorders, heart disease, headaches and migraines, fibromyalgia, alcohol addiction, digestion, gut problems, memory problems, mood disorders, MS, and even cancer.

There are many recorded ways to activate the nerve of the vagus, such as singing and humming, laughing, yoga, mindfulness, breathing exercises, physical activity, and vibration, just to name a few. Singing and smiling activates the muscles that trigger the nerve at the back of your throat. In addition, mild exercise or rehabilitation raises the blood of the stomach, which means the nerve of the vagus is activated. Owing to the motions, a regimented yoga practise can also improve this nerve's activation, but relaxation and OM-ing do help stimulate the vagus nerve. All these ways the vagus nerve can be activated have one thing in common: tone!!

"Stress and disease cause interacting neural circuits in which interleukin-1 as a mediator is critically involved," Maier said.

However, not only does stress produce the predicted response to stress, it also causes precisely the same behavioral changes— including reduced intake of food however water and decreased exploration— and physiological changes, including temperature, elevated white blood cell counts, and active macrophages seen in the "sickness response," Maier said. "You see all the infection you see." What does that mean to you? "Stress is a different kind of disease," Maier said. "And the effects of anxiety are... the stimulation of receptors that have naturally developed to protect against disease." So, the next time you feel "sick," you're going to have stress as a cause. The boss who stresses you when you see them, listen to their voice or even receive an email from them. The pressure to perform and you're not sure you can get the job done when you are asked to take on a new role or task that you either feel unqualified or are not prepared to do. Of course, if you seem likely to lose your job, the stress level will rise dramatically!

Bear in mind that stress can also play a role with others. If your partner or other important other is ill, you must understand the burden they may have had before they get sick. For example, if your kids are sick on an ongoing basis, it could be a sign that somewhere in their life, there is ongoing pressure. I don't assume that all illness is related to stress, but there's an explanation we've got what's called "dis-ease." Dream about it.

IMPORTANCE OF THE VAGUS NERVE FOR HEALTH AND WEIGHT LOSS

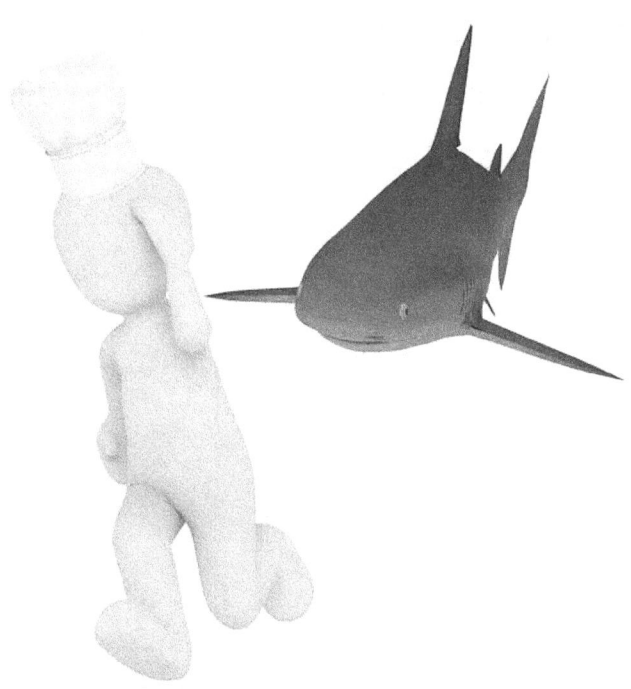

The Most Important Nerve you Didn't Know you Had

Have you ever wondered why, after consuming a small amount of food, some people feel satisfied, and others are still hungry before they eat a big meal?

The response may be in their vagus nerve's responsiveness. The vagus nerve is the nerve that binds your stomach to your brain, and it is an important part of the parasympathetic nervous system (the "rest and eat" response, literally the "fight or flight" opposite).

Signals from the intestine to the brain running up the vagus nerve affect your perception of hunger and fullness, your mood and stress levels, and your response to inflammatory stress.

Signals running down the vagus nerve from the brain to the gut impact absorption, digestive enzyme production, and gastrointestinal motility (this is a fancy word on the spectrum of constipation to diarrhea).

It is a very important pathway, and vagus nerve activation involves obesity, gastrointestinal diseases, cardiovascular diseases, mood disorders such as depression, and all sorts of other chronic health issues. Here is a look at why the vagus nerve is so important and how your diet can improve your wellbeing by influencing vagal nerve signals from the intestine.

The Vagus Nerve Controls How Hungry you Feel

Hunger and fullness signals are an essential form of interaction that flows up and down the vagus nerve. For examples:

- The actual mass of belly food gives satiety signals to your brain from the vagus nerve. This is how the brain knows that after a meal you can stop feeling thirsty.
- Sensors of nutrients and neurotransmitters released in the intestine, such as serotonin and ghrelin, may also send signals of hunger and fullness to the brain.

Obesity is associated with a lower sensitivity of the vagus nerve to signals of fullness, and there is a lot of evidence that this is caused by diet in particular. Obesity-inducing diets can change the sensitivity of the vagus nerve to fullness signals, so getting the "full now" signal takes more food for your brain. And as you might expect, stimulating the vagus nerve (to "turn the volume" on the satiety signal) in experimental animals tends to cause weight loss–although it is worth noting that human studies have mixed results.

Vagus Nerve and Other Health Issues

Hunger is a major reason why the nerve of the vagus is important. But if you dive PubMed, you will find that vagus nerve dysfunction is associated with other problems of all kinds. That's because the vagus nerve also helps regulate inflammation, and just about every chronic disease involves inflammation. Anti-inflammatory is the activation of vagus nerve impulses to the brain–this allows the brain to turn down the stress response and reduce the production of inflammatory cytokines.

The effects here are a bit difficult to untangle because the vagus nerve is a two-way street, and there are a lot of complicated feedback loops between the brain and the intestine (remember the vagus nerve runs both ways!). But the exact mechanism may be less important for people who are just concerned about improving their health:

- Inflammation control of the vagus nerve affects cardiovascular health, and stimulation of the vagus nerve can help prevent cardiovascular events.
- Vagus nerve signaling is discarded in Crohn's disease patients (a form of inflammatory intestinal disease), and a small preliminary study found that vagal nerve stimulation helps to treat the symptoms.
- Irritable bowel syndrome may also affect the vagus nerve, and vagal stimulation may help reduce IBS pain.
- This experiment is really interesting: both anxiety and insulin resistance is avoided by treating diabetes-prone rats with vagal nerve stimulation. This is an important piece of evidence that both anxiety and diabetes may have origins in the stomach.

If a bad diet affects the vagus nerve's resistance, it may also cause all of these diseases in the second hand. It could be one explanation why in overall health, gut health is such a big player.

Care and Feeding of your Vagus Nerve

So far, we know that an obesogenic "cafeteria diet" (high-fat, high-carb junk food) reduces the vagus nerve's sensitivity and that vagus nerve stimulation counteracts that, with great weight benefits... and just about everything else. Unfortunately, in these studies, "vagal nerve stimulation" is not something that you can do at home; it is a device that has been surgically implanted in their bodies by the subjects.

But the vagus nerve's sensitivity can be reduced by a lousy diet, and perhaps a good diet can help restore it. Apart from "don't eat a diet of junk food," here is a bit more specific research.

This study found inflammation decreased by dietary fat through its effects on the nerve of the vagus. The authors concluded that "high-fat... nutrition is potentially beneficial in multiple inflammatory disorders such as sepsis and inflammatory bowel disease (IBD) caused by an inflammatory response in which... intestinal barrier function is compromised." This is confirmed by the link between a ketogenic (very high-fat, low-carb) diet and vagal nerve stimulation. A ketogenic diet may have some of its anti-inflammatory effects that suppress hunger by stimulating the vagus nerve.

This study also found that the vagus nerve had been activated by a probiotic (Lactobacillus casei strain Shirota). For students taking a traumatic test, the probiotic changed the gut-to-brain pressure signaling and reduced the release of the stress hormone cortisol. It suggests that probiotics could break the cycle of gut-brain-gut-brain feedback up and down the vagus nerve, where psychological stress causes trouble in the gut, which sends more signals of hormonal stress to the brain, causing more trouble in the gut.

You can also use the Valsalva maneuver to conduct your vagal nerve stimulation for instant gratification. Sit down, and it can make you somewhat dizzy. Take a deep breath, then open the eyes and pinch the nose so that no wind can escape. Then say you're trying to breathe in, but you should feel the pressure from the wind without opening your nose or mouth. Try to do this for 15-20 seconds, and then let the water out and breathe normally. (If you d o any weightlifting, this is the kind of breath-holding that you do to balance your back during hard squats or deadlifts.) The Valsa maneuver does not have long-term effects, but it may be useful for an immediate situation, just before an exam or in the midst of a tense flow.

That's not much to go on with –there are not a lot of food or vagus nerve trials. But starting with it is something, and it reinforces the important ways that the gut, the brain, and the rest of your body are all connected. Understanding the vagus nerve helps explain why digestive health, mental health, and the health of the whole body are so intertwined with each other, and why good gut health is so critical for issues that go well beyond digestion.

CONCLUSIONS

One of the keys to dealing with anxiety is to learn how through proper breathing to stimulate your vagus nerve. The vagus nerve serves as the bridge between the mind and the body and regulates the reaction to relax. When performing diaphragmatic breathing with the partially closed glottis, you will relax the vagus nerve. Use your dead time to regularly use this technique, turn it into a routine, and the effects will amaze you.

The vagus nerve is the parasympathetic nervous system's most important element (the one that calms you down by controlling your response to relaxation).

It originates from the brainstem and is "wandering" all the way down into the abdomen, extending fibers to the tongue, pharynx, vocal chords, lungs, chest, liver, intestines, and glands releasing anti-stress enzymes and hormones (such as acetylcholine, prolactin, vasopressin, oxytocin), affecting appetite, metabolism and, of course, the calming reaction.

Vagus nerve acts as the connection between the mind and the body, and it is the cable behind the emotions and intestinal instincts of your heart. The key to managing your mental state and levels of anxiety can activate your parasympathetic system's calming nervous pathways.

This part of the nervous system cannot be managed on request, but you can partially activate the vagus nerve by:

- Immerse your head in cold water (diving reflex)
- Trying to exhale against a blocked airway (Valsalva maneuver).
- You can do this by holding your mouth shut and pinching your nose while trying to breathe out. It greatly increases the tension

inside the chest cavity relaxing the vagus nerve and increasing vagal tone
- Singing

And of course, diaphragmatic breathing exercises Strengthening it living nervous system will pay great dividends, and the best tool to do this is by exercising the body.

REFERENCES

1. ^ Dutchman M, Bautista TG, Mörschel M, Dick TE (May 2014). "Learning to breathe: habituation of Hering-Breuer inflation reflex emerges with postnatal brainstem maturation". Respiratory Physiology & Neurobiology. 195: 44–9. doi: 10.1016/j.resp.2014.02.009. PMC 4111629. PMID 24566392.
2. 2. ^ Eljamel, Sam (2011). Problem Based Neurosurgery. p. 66. doi: 10.1142/7830. ISBN 978-981-4317-07-8.
3. 3. ^ Mandal, Ananya (25 September 2013). "Vomiting Mechanism". News Medical. Archived from the original on 4 January 2015. Retrieved 27 June 2015.
4. 4. ^ Berthoud HR (August 2008). "The vagus nerve, food intake and obesity". Regulatory Peptides. 149 (1–3): 15–25. doi: 10.1016/j.re.gpep.2007.08.024. PMC 2597723. PMID 18482776.
5. 5. ^ de Lartigue G, Ronveaux CC, Raybould HE (September 2014). "Deletion of leptin signaling in vagal afferent neurons results in hyperphagia and obesity". Molecular Metabolism. 3 (6): 595–607. doi: 10.1016/j.molmet.2014.06.003. PMC 4142400. PMID 25161883.
6. 6. ^ "Exploring the Mind-Body Orgasm". Wired. 10 January 2007. Archived from the original on 19 September 2015.
7. 7. ^ Pocai A, Lam TK, Gutierrez-Juarez R, Obici S,
8. Schwartz GJ, Bryan J, Aguilar-Bryan L, Rossetti L (April 2005). "Hypothalamic K (ATP) channels control hepatic glucose production". Nature. 434 (7036): 1026–31. doi: 10.1038/nature03439. PMID 15846348.

www.ingramcontent.com/pod-product-compliance
Lightning Source LLC
Chambersburg PA
CBHW070624220526
45466CB00001B/90